Infectious Disease

Editor

ROBERT PAXTON

PHYSICIAN ASSISTANT CLINICS

www.physicianassistant.theclinics.com

Consulting Editor
JAMES A. VAN RHEE

April 2017 • Volume 2 • Number 2

ELSEVIER

1600 John F. Kennedy Boulevard • Suite 1800 • Philadelphia, Pennsylvania, 19103-2899

http://www.theclinics.com

PHYSICIAN ASSISTANT CLINICS Volume 2, Number 2
April 2017 ISSN 2405-7991, ISBN-13: 978-0-323-52425-4

Editor: Jessica McCool
Developmental Editor: Casey Potter

Physician Assistant Clinics (ISSN: 2405–7991) is published quarterly by Elsevier Inc., 360 Park Avenue South, New York, NY 10010-1710. Months of issue are January, April, July, and October. Periodicals postage paid at New York, NY and additional mailing offices. Subscription prices are $150.00 per year (US individuals), $205.00 (US institutions), $100.00 (US students), $210.00 (Canadian individuals), $257.00 (Canadian institutions), $100.00 (Canadian students), $150.00 (international individuals), $257.00 (international institutions), and $100.00 (international students). Foreign air speed delivery is included in all *Clinics* subscription prices. All prices are subject to change without notice. POSTMASTER: Send address changes to *Physician Assistant Clinics*, Elsevier Periodicals Customer Service, 11830 Westline Industrial Drive, St. Louis, MO 63146. Customer Service Health Sciences Division, Subscription Customer Service, 3251 Riverport Lane, Maryland Heights, MO 63043. **Customer Service: 1-800-654-2452 (U.S. and Canada); 314-447-8871 (outside U.S. and Canada). Fax: 314-447-8029. E-mail:** journalscustomerservice-usa@elsevier.com **(for print support);** journalsonlinesupport-usa@elsevier.com **(for online support).**

Reprints. For copies of 100 or more, of articles in this publication, please contact the Commercial Reprints Department, Elsevier Inc., 360 Park Avenue South, New York, NY 10010-1710. Tel. 212-633-3874; Fax: 212-633-3820; E-mail: reprints@elsevier.com.

Physician Assistant Clinics is covered in *MEDLINE/PubMed (Index Medicus)* and *EMBASE/Excerpta Medica, Current Contents/Clinical Medicine, and ISI/BIOMED.*

PROGRAM OBJECTIVE
The goal of the Physician Assistant Clinics is to keep practicing physician assistants up to date with current clinical practice by providing timely articles reviewing the state of the art in patient care.

TARGET AUDIENCE
Physician Assistants and other healthcare professionals.

LEARNING OBJECTIVES
Upon completion of this activity, participants will be able to:
1. Review updates on treatments for infectious diseases including human immunodeficiency virus, sexually transmitted infections, and hepatitis C.
2. Discuss the management of infectious diseases such as mycobacterium tuberculosis, bite wounds, and mononucleosis.
3. Recognize the management of common infections such as tickborne infections, infectious diarrhea, and endemic fungal infections, among others.

ACCREDITATION
The Elsevier Office of Continuing Medical Education (EOCME) is accredited by the Accreditation Council for Continuing Medical Education (ACCME) to provide continuing medical education for physicians.

The EOCME designates this enduring material for a maximum of 15 *AMA PRA Category 1 Credit*(s)™. Physicians should claim only the credit commensurate with the extent of their participation in the activity.

All other health care professionals requesting continuing education credit for this enduring material will be issued a certificate of participation.

DISCLOSURE OF CONFLICTS OF INTEREST
The EOCME assesses conflict of interest with its instructors, faculty, planners, and other individuals who are in a position to control the content of CME activities. All relevant conflicts of interest that are identified are thoroughly vetted by EOCME for fair balance, scientific objectivity, and patient care recommendations. EOCME is committed to providing its learners with CME activities that promote improvements or quality in healthcare and not a specific proprietary business or a commercial interest.

The planning committee, staff, authors and editors listed below have identified no financial relationships or relationships to products or devices they or their spouse/life partner have with commercial interest related to the content of this CME activity:
Kartikey Acharya, MD, MPH; Kathleen M. Barta, PA-C, MPAS; Roy A. Borchardt, PA-C, PhD; Mary Broadhurst, PA-C, MPAS; Joseph Daniel; Erin DuHaime, PA-C; Ronald W. Flenner, MD; Anjali Fortna; Nancy Ivansek, PA-C, MA; Casey Potter; Patricia R. Jennings, PA-C, DrPH; Kyle Kalchbrenner, PA-C, MPAS; Stephanie L. Ludtke, PA-C, MPAS; Jessica McCool; Karen McMenemy, RPA-C, MS; Robert Paxton, PA-C, MPAS; Christopher Roman, PA-C, MA, MMS; Terry Scott, PA-C, MPA, DFAAPA; Jamie R. Silkey, PA-C, MPAS, MHA; Tia Solh, PA-C, MT(ASCP), MPAS; Susan Sweeney Stewart, PA-C, MPH, MMSc; Susan Symington, PA-C, MPAS, DFAAPA; Rebekah Thomas, PA-C, PharmD, BCPS, BC-ADM; Michelle Touw, PA-C, MMS; James A. Van Rhee, PA-C, MS; Katie Widmeier; Amy Williams; Leah Hampson Yoke, PA-C, MCHS.

UNAPPROVED/OFF-LABEL USE DISCLOSURE
The EOCME requires CME faculty to disclose to the participants:
1. When products or procedures being discussed are off-label, unlabelled, experimental, and/or investigational (not US Food and Drug Administration [FDA] approved); and
2. Any limitations on the information presented, such as data that are preliminary or that represent ongoing research, interim analyses, and/or unsupported opinions. Faculty may discuss information about pharmaceutical agents that is outside of FDA-approved labelling. This information is intended solely for CME and is not intended to promote off-label use of these medications. If you have any questions, contact the medical affairs department of the manufacturer for the most recent prescribing information.

TO ENROLL
The CME program is available to all Physician Assistant Clinics subscribers at no additional fee. To subscribe to the Physician Assistant Clinics, call customer service at 1-800-654-2452 or sign up online at www.physicianassistant.theclinics.com.

METHOD OF PARTICIPATION

In order to claim credit, participants must complete the following:

1. Complete enrolment as indicated above.
2. Read the activity.
3. Complete the CME Test and Evaluation. Participants must achieve a score of 70% on the test. All CME Tests and Evaluations must be completed online.

CME INQUIRIES/SPECIAL NEEDS

For all CME inquiries or special needs, please contact elsevierCME@elsevier.com.

Contributors

CONSULTING EDITOR

JAMES A. VAN RHEE, PA-C, MS
Associate Professor, Program Director, Yale School of Medicine, Yale Physician Assistant
Online Program, New Haven, Connecticut

EDITOR

ROBERT PAXTON, PA-C, MPAS
Associate Department Chair & Director of Didactic Education, Clinical Associate
Professor, Department of Physician Assistant Studies, Marquette University, Milwaukee,
Wisconsin

AUTHORS

KARTIKEY ACHARYA, MD, MPH
Assistant Professor of Medicine, Division of Infectious Diseases, Medical College of
Wisconsin, Milwaukee, Wisconsin

KATHLEEN M. BARTA, PA-C, MPAS
Infectious Diseases Specialists of Southeastern Wisconsin, Brookfield, Wisconsin

ROY A. BORCHARDT, PA-C, PhD
Physician Assistant and Supervisor, Advanced Practice Providers, Department of
Infectious Diseases, Infection Control and Employee Health, MD Anderson Cancer Center,
Houston, Texas

MARY BROADHURST, PA-C, MPAS
Department of Infectious Diseases, Saint Vincent Hospital, Indianapolis, Indiana

ERIN DuHAIME, PA-C
Physician Assistant Certified, Infectious Diseases, Baylor University Medical Center,
Dallas, Texas

RONALD W. FLENNER, MD
Vice Dean, Academic Affairs, Eastern Virginia Medical School, Norfolk, Virginia

NANCY IVANSEK, PA-C, MA
Director, Clinical Curriculum, Physician Assistant Program, Case Western Reserve
University; Physician Assistant, Infectious Disease Department, Cleveland Clinic
Foundation, Cleveland, Ohio

PATRICIA R. JENNINGS, PA-C, DrPH
Professor, Eastern Virginia Medical School, Norfolk, Virginia

KYLE KALCHBRENNER, PA-C, MPAS
Physician Assistant specializing in Infectious Diseases, Burr Ridge, Illinois

STEPHANIE L. LUDTKE, PA-C, MPAS
Physician Assistant, Division of Joint Reconstruction, Department of Orthopaedic
Surgery, Medical College of Wisconsin, Milwaukee, Wisconsin

KAREN McMENEMY, RPA-C, MS
Department of Medicine, NYU-Lutheran Medical Center, Brooklyn, New York

CHRISTOPHER ROMAN, PA-C, MA, MMS
Assistant Professor, Department of Physician Assistant Studies, Butler University,
Indianapolis, Indiana

TERRY SCOTT, PA-C, MPA, DFAAPA
Assistant Professor; Program Director/Section Head, MEDEX Northwest PA Program,
Department of Family Medicine, University of Washington, Seattle, Washington

JAMIE R. SILKEY, PA-C, MPAS, MHA
Physician Assistant, Division of Foot and Ankle Surgery, Department of Orthopaedic
Surgery, Medical College of Wisconsin, Milwaukee, Wisconsin

TIA SOLH, PA-C, MT(ASCP), MPAS
Clinical Assistant Professor, Department of Physician Assistant Studies, Mercer
University, Atlanta, Georgia

SUSAN SWEENEY STEWART, PA-C, MPH, MMSc
Atlanta ID Group, Atlanta, Georgia

SUSAN SYMINGTON, PA-C, MPAS, DFAAPA
Associate Professor; Associate Program Director, MEDEX Northwest PA Program,
Department of Family Medicine, University of Washington, Seattle, Washington

REBEKAH THOMAS, PA-C, PharmD, BCPS, BC-ADM
Department of Physician Assistant Studies, Philadelphia College of Osteopathic
Medicine, Suwanee, Georgia

MICHELLE TOUW, PA-C, MMS
Division of Infectious Diseases, Department of Internal Medicine, Eastern Virginia Medical
School, Norfolk, Virginia

LEAH HAMPSON YOKE, PA-C, MCHS
Vaccine and Infectious Disease Division, Fred Hutchinson Cancer Research Center;
Allergy and Infectious Disease Division, University of Washington School of Medicine,
Seattle, Washington

Contents

Foreword: The Physician Assistant: Fifty Years of Patient Care   xiii

James A. Van Rhee

Preface: Physician Assistants' Role in Twenty-First Century Infectious Diseases   xv

Robert Paxton

**Community-Acquired Pneumonia: Making Use of the Guidelines from Pediatrics
to Adults**   155

Susan Symington and Terry Scott

> Community-acquired pneumonia (CAP) is a common illness with a high
> mortality rate throughout the world. It affects patients of all ages. Prac-
> ticing in a primary care setting requires knowledge, diagnostic skills, and
> treatments that are recommended to prevent, improve outcomes, and
> also reduce the incidence of antibiotic resistance to common pathogens
> that cause CAP. Guidelines from the American and British Thoracic Soci-
> eties and also the Pediatric and Adult Infectious Diseases of American So-
> cieties have published guidelines for clinicians to follow. This article
> summarizes the current published guidelines for the management and
> treatment of CAP.

Skin and Soft Tissue Infections   165

Karen McMenemy

> Skin and soft tissue infections are among the most commonly encoun-
> tered, and run the continuum from mild to life-threatening. In the last
> three decades, emerging resistance patterns in common pathogens
> have drastically increased morbidity and mortality of the affected pa-
> tients, and caused a rapid increase in health care utilization. By strati-
> fying patient risk factors and becoming familiar with epidemiology of
> these infections, we can focus treatment plans and improve patient
> outcomes.

Key Points Review of Meningitis   177

Susan Sweeney Stewart

> Meningitis is a serious illness, particularly bacterial meningitis, and usually
> is easy to diagnose with the aid of a complete history and physical exam-
> ination. Ninety-five percent of persons with bacterial meningitis present
> with 2 of the following 4 symptoms: fever, nuchal rigidity, altered mental
> status, or headache. However, viral meningitis is far more common. The
> diagnostic dilemma of determining the etiologic agent can be tricky de-
> pending on a person's age, past medical history (eg, immunosuppression),
> and other risk factors, but this should not cause a delay in administration of
> empiric antibiotics.

Current Diagnosis and Management of Urinary Tract Infections   191

Tia Solh, Rebekah Thomas, and Christopher Roman

Urinary tract infections (UTIs) are commonly encountered bacterial infections, and knowledge of current diagnosis and management is vital. Diagnosis of UTIs relies on history and physical examination, evaluation of risk factors, and urinalysis results. Escherichia coli remains the most frequent cause of UTIs, but rising antimicrobial resistance has changed the landscape of treatment. Practitioners must be familiar with local resistance patterns when prescribing and must be able to distinguish UTIs from asymptomatic bacteriuria and candiduria to prevent further antimicrobial resistance. This article reviews the epidemiology, risk factors, pathophysiology, and current diagnosis and treatment of UTIs.

Sexually Transmitted Infections: A Medical Update   207

Patricia R. Jennings and Ronald W. Flenner

The term sexually transmitted infections (STIs) refers to a variety of clinical syndromes and infections caused by pathogens that can be acquired and transmitted through sexual activity. The CDC estimates that nearly 20 million new STIs occur every year in this country and account for almost $16 billion in health care costs. Physician assistants (PAs) play a critical role in identifying, treating, and preventing STIs. As part of the clinical encounter, PAs should routinely obtain sexual histories from patients and address risk reduction. This article reviews recent demographics and current screening, diagnostic testing, and treatment of common STIs.

An Overview of Best Practice Guidelines for *Mycobacterium tuberculosis* Screening and Treatment   219

Nancy Ivansek

The elimination of tuberculosis (TB) in the United States is greatly dependent on health care providers being knowledgeable about current guidelines for TB screening and the appropriate treatment of active and latent disease. The identification and treatment of active tuberculosis is the most important reason for screening for *Mycobacterium tuberculosis*. Screening for latent TB also has an important place in public health, disease management, and reducing the potential sources of infection. This article discusses the importance of screening, the current recommendations for choosing a screening test, and presents an overview of current treatment guidelines for both active and latent disease.

Infectious Diarrhea   229

Christopher Roman, Tia Solh, and Mary Broadhurst

Infectious diarrhea is a common problem with a tremendous domestic and global burden of disease. Most cases of diarrhea are benign and self-limited, but several pathogens are important because of their frequency and/or severity. The fundamental characteristics of several such diseases are considered in this review, along with current recommendations for diagnosis and treatment. The pathogens discussed are norovirus, *Campylobacter*, *Salmonella* (typhoid and nontyphoid), *Shigella*, Shiga toxin–producing *Escherichia coli*, *Giardia*, and *Cryptosporidium*.

Tickborne Infections 247

Kathleen M. Barta

> Tickborne infections are prevalent in many areas of the United States and presentation varies widely. Diagnosis can be challenging and is easily missed if tick bite, travel, and environmental history is not asked. Coinfection with 2 or more tickborne infections is rare but can be seen. This article reviews the most common tickborne infections in the United States. The etiology, clinical manifestations, diagnostic testing, and therapeutic treatments based on the most current recommendations are reviewed. In addition, when to treat empirically and the use of antibiotics in adults and pediatric populations is covered.

Orthopedic Infections 261

Jamie R. Silkey, Stephanie L. Ludtke, and Kartikey Acharya

> Orthopedic infections vary in presentation and pathophysiology. This article reviews the etiology, pathophysiology, clinical manifestations, diagnostic testing, and treatment options for infectious arthritis of native joints and osteomyelitis. Systemic factors in patients with diabetes and vascular disease make them vulnerable to these infections. Diagnostic testing can assist in making an accurate diagnosis and ruling out differential diagnoses. Antibiotic therapy is guided by culture and sensitivity results, but occasionally empiric therapy is required when cultures are unavailable or altered by previous antibiotic usage. Diagnosis, treatment, and management of orthopedic infections require multidisciplinary collaboration between infectious disease, orthopedic surgery, and radiology.

Managing Common Bite Wounds and Their Complications in the United States 277

Kyle Kalchbrenner

> Bite wounds are common in the United States and are frequently caused by dogs, cats, and other humans. Although the likelihood of rabies transmission from these organisms is low in this region of the world, the risk of infection is high. Wounds must be thoroughly cleaned, evaluated, and documented for signs of complication. After workup, it is important to begin broad-spectrum antimicrobial therapy, including coverage for *Pasteurella* and *Eikenella,* and including further gram-positive, gram-negative, and anaerobic coverage. This article will help the clinician through this seemingly simple, but often-complicated process to ensure the patient is receiving exceptional care.

A Tale of Two Mononucleosis Syndromes: Cytomegalovirus and Epstein-Barr Virus for the Primary Care Provider 287

Leah Hampson Yoke

> Cytomegalovirus and Epstein-Barr virus are 2 herpesviruses that can cause mononucleosis syndromes in immunocompetent patients. These syndromes are challenging to diagnose and manage but can be common in primary care settings. Here we review these viruses while providing a helpful framework for the clinician to order laboratory tests, evaluate alternative diagnoses, and treat patients in an evidence-based manner.

Endemic Fungal Infections in the United States   297

Roy A. Borchardt

In the United States, *Blastomyces dermatitidis*, *Coccidioides* spp, and *Histoplasma capsulatum*, primarily cause endemic mycoses and are frequently overlooked as causes of community acquired pneumonia. Most commonly presenting as pneumonia, they can progress to disease in various tissues, including the central nervous system. Diagnosis is made by microorganism culture from respiratory or tissue cultures. Serologic testing can aid in the diagnosis but crossover reactivity is significant. Polymerase chain reaction testing is available. Antifungal azoles and amphotericin B formulations are the preferred drugs. Treatment typically requires extended antifungal therapy. The Infectious Diseases Society of America offers recommendations.

Hepatitis C: An Update on Next Generation Treatment and Clinical Cure   313

Erin DuHaime

Hepatitis C is an important chronic infectious disease that primarily infects hepatocytes causing progressive liver disease. An estimated 3 to 4 million people in the United States and 170 million people in the world have chronic hepatitis C disease, and a large number remain undiagnosed. Screening recommendations are generally based on age and risk factors, and once diagnosed with hepatitis C, most patients are eligible for treatment. With the introduction of new antiviral therapies for hepatitis C virus, there are regimens with markedly improved tolerability, dosing schedules, and efficacy approaching 100% for all genotypes.

Update on Human Immunodeficiency Virus   327

Michelle Touw

Human immunodeficiency virus (HIV) continues to spread worldwide. In at-risk populations in the United States, only 25% of people living with HIV attend care regularly and have full viral suppression. At-risk individuals should be screened frequently, and new fourth-generation tests may be positive as early as 3 weeks after infection and during acute retroviral syndrome. Major public health efforts are focused on identifying at-risk individuals, testing and treating positive patients, and providing pre-exposure prophylaxis when appropriate. Newer antiretroviral regimens are very effective and tolerable with many single-tablet regimens and once-daily options.

PHYSICIAN ASSISTANT CLINICS

FORTHCOMING ISSUES

July 2017
Emergency Medicine
Fred Wu and Michael E. Winters, *Editors*

October 2017
Cardiology
Daniel Thibodeau, *Editor*

January 2018
Urology
Todd J. Doran, *Editor*

RECENT ISSUES

January 2017
Endocrinology
Ji Hyun Chun (CJ), *Editor*

October 2016
Pediatrics
Kristyn Lowery, Brian Wingrove, and
Genevieve A.N. DelRosario, *Editors*

July 2016
Oncology
Alexandria Garino, *Editor*

RELATED INTEREST

Infectious Disease Clinics of North America
September 2016 (Vol. 30, Issue 3)
**Infection Prevention and Control in Healthcare, Part 1: Facility Planning and
Management**
Keith S. Kaye and Sorabh Dhar, *Editors*

Infectious Disease Clinics of North America
December 2016 (Vol. 30, Issue 4)
**Infection Prevention and Control in Healthcare, Part II: Epidemiology and Prevention
of Infections**
Keith S. Kaye and Sorabh Dhar, *Editors*

THE CLINICS ARE AVAILABLE ONLINE!
Access your subscription at:
www.theclinics.com

FORTHCOMING ISSUES

July 2017
Endocrinology
Fred J. Wu and Michael J. Wolfen, Editors

October 2017
Cardiology
Daniel T. Thibodeau, Editor

January 2018
Urology
Todd J. Doran, Editor

RECENT ISSUES

January 2017
Endocrinology
Fred J. Wu and Michael Gooch, Editor

October 2016
Pediatrics
Kristyn Lowery, Susan Wanamaker, and
Genevieve A.N. DelRosario, Editors

July 2016
Oncology
Alexandria Garino, Editor

RELATED INTEREST

Infectious Disease Clinics of North America
September 2016 (Vol. 30, Issue 3)
Infection Prevention and Control in Healthcare, Part I: Facility Planning and
Management
Keith S. Kaye and Joseph Obbi, Editors

Infectious Disease Clinics of North America
December 2016 (Vol. 30, Issue 4)
Infection Prevention and Control in Healthcare, Part II: Epidemiology and Prevention
of Infections
Keith S. Kaye and Sorabh Dhar, Editors

Foreword

The Physician Assistant: Fifty Years of Patient Care

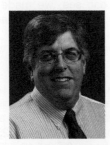

James A. Van Rhee, PA-C, MS
Consulting Editor

It has been fifty years since the first "Physician's Assistant" (yes, the apostrophe was left in on purpose to remind us how far we have come) class graduated at Duke in 1967. From that first class of 3 graduates, we now have over 108,000 certified physician assistants in the United States. We all know about the efforts of Dr Eugene Stead in bringing the physician assistant profession to fruition, but how many of us recognize the names of Eugene Schneller, Barbara Andrew, Thomas Piemme, Hu Myers, Edward Pellegrino, and Alfred Sadler? I was very fortunate to sit down with Dr Alfred Sadler,[1] founder and director of the Yale PA Program and first president of the Association of Physician Assistant Programs, now known as the Physician Assistant Education Association, a few weeks ago to talk about the history of the PA profession. During that time, we talked about the start of the profession, the development of the educational programs, development of the PA practice act, the first board examination, and the growth of the PA profession over these fifty years. Talking to Dr Sadler, a person on the ground and in the trenches during this time, provided me with new insight into the profession that I thought I understood. I would strongly encourage every PA to visit the Physician Assistant History Society website at http://www.pahx.org to find out about our early leaders as we as a profession look to our future and all the changes we are facing.

Enough about the past, let's talk about the present and this issue of *Physician Assistant Clinics*. In this issue, we focus on infectious diseases. While we have an excellent update on HIV by Touw, Robert Paxton, PA-C, MPAS, the guest editor of this issue, made a concerted effort to make sure this issue covered more than just HIV. In this issue, we cover infectious disease in just about every organ system. We have Symington and Scott providing us with an excellent review of community-acquired pneumonia and Ivansek providing a review on best practice guidelines on tuberculosis, so we have the pulmonary system covered. We have the skin covered with two articles: McMenemy with skin and soft tissue infections and Kalchbrenner on managing bite wounds and their complications. In the gastrointestinal system, Roman, Ludtke, and Acharya

Physician Assist Clin 2 (2017) xiii–xiv
http://dx.doi.org/10.1016/j.cpha.2017.01.002
2405-7991/17/

provide us with a review of infectious diarrhea, and DuHaime reviews hepatitis C. Solh, Thomas, and Roman cover urinary tract infections, and Jennings provides an update on sexually transmitted infections, so we have the genitourinary tract covered. The neurologic system is covered by Stewart with her review of meningitis. Silkey, Ludtke, and Acharya cover orthopedic infections. And, to round it out with miscellanea, we have Barta covering tick-borne infections, Yoke covering mononucleosis syndromes, and Borchardt covering endemic fungal infections. As you can see, we made a conscious effort to represent infectious diseases that plague (pun intended) nearly every organ system in the human body.

I hope you enjoy the sixth issue of *Physician Assistant Clinics*. Our next issue will provide a review of the latest in emergency medicine.

James A. Van Rhee, PA-C, MS
Yale School of Medicine
Yale Physician Assistant Online Program
100 Church Street South, Suite A250
New Haven, CT 06519, USA

E-mail addresses:
james.vanrhee@yale.edu
Website: http://www.paonline.yale.edu

REFERENCE

1. Physician Assistant History Society, Johns Creek, GA. Biography, Sadler, Alfred M. Available at: http://www.pahx.org/sadler-alfred-m. Accessed January 4, 2017.

Preface

Physician Assistants' Role in Twenty-First Century Infectious Diseases

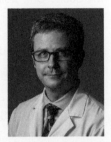

Robert Paxton, PA-C, MPAS
Editor

Infectious diseases are frequently encountered entities, but frequently misunderstood because of various etiologies, multiple and often overlapping presentations, and a panoply of diagnostic and treatment modalities. These diseases also provoke emotional responses in patients that are different than many other clinical conditions. Compounding this is the constant addition of newly "discovered" infections. New infectious disease entities seem to be in the news on a regular basis. As evidenced by the recent global fear surrounding the Ebola outbreak in West Africa in 2014 and Zika virus potentially impacting the Olympics. In addition to these widely reported diseases, we have Chikungunya virus, pandemic *C difficile*, drug-resistant *Enterobacteriaceae*, Middle East Respiratory Syndrome Coronavirus, community-acquired *Staphylococcus aureus*, various tick-borne diseases, and many others.

The development of this issue is wide ranging with nearly every major organ system being represented. While you will find several of the topics familiar, there are also updates on infections that have transitioned as diseases that will be managed more frequently in the future by physician assistants. As an example, progressive medical updates regarding human immunodeficiency virus (HIV) and hepatitis C virus (HCV) now have significant implications for both primary and specialty physician assistants. From the dramatic change in pharmacologic options over the last few years for HCV to pre-exposure prophylaxis for HIV, physician assistants are now on the frontline of patient management for these infectious diseases.

While many infectious diseases are encountered and managed by the primary care provider, many infectious diseases are optimally managed as part of a team with an infectious disease specialist. A recent study has demonstrated infectious disease consultation with lower health care costs and mortality.[1] In this issue of *Physician Assistant Clinics,* there are wonderful medical updates by specialists throughout the

Physician Assist Clin 2 (2017) xv–xvi
http://dx.doi.org/10.1016/j.cpha.2017.01.001
2405-7991/17/© 2017 Elsevier Inc. All rights reserved.

physicianassistant.theclinics.com

country. I hope this issue illustrates the significant contribution physician assistants have made in the management of infectious diseases.

I would like to thank the *Physician Assistant Clinics* consulting editor, James A. Van Rhee, PA-C for inviting me to develop this issue and for the assistance from the editorial staff. I hope you enjoy reading this journal as much as I did developing it.

Robert Paxton, PA-C, MPAS
Department of Physician Assistant Studies
Marquette University
Milwaukee, WI 53201-1881, USA

E-mail address:
Robert.paxton@marquette.edu

REFERENCE

1. Schmitt S, McQuillen DP, Nahass R, et al. Infectious diseases specialty intervention is associated with decreased mortality and lower healthcare costs. Clin Infect Dis 2014;58(1):22–8.

Community-Acquired Pneumonia

Making Use of the Guidelines from Pediatrics to Adults

Susan Symington, PA-C, MPAS, DFAAPA*, Terry Scott, PA-C, MPA, DFAAPA

KEYWORDS

- Community acquired pneumonia (CAP) • Infectious disease • Pediatric • Adult
- Health prevention

KEY POINTS

- Community-acquired pneumonia continues to be a common illness and cause of death in the world.
- Prevention of CAP is key to reduce the incidence of *Streptococcus pneumoniae* types that are increasingly becoming resistant to antibiotic therapy.
- In clinical practice, it is important to follow the established guidelines published by the British and American Thoracic Societies and the Infectious Diseases Societies of America.

INTRODUCTION

Community-acquired pneumonia (CAP) is a leading cause of illness and mortality in the world. It is a condition that is underdiagnosed and undertreated.[1–3] Providers should follow the recommended guidelines that have been established recently for the management and treatment of CAP in both children and adults. The guidelines for the management and treatment of CAP have been established by the American and British Thoracic Societies, as well as the Infectious Diseases Society of America.[3–5] Unfortunately, antibiotic resistance is steadily increasing, which complicates proper treatment.[6] This article summarizes the pediatric and adult guidelines and focuses on outpatient treatment and when it is most appropriate to admit a patient with CAP to the hospital.

CAP is defined as pneumonia that is contracted by an individual within a community and is not to be confused with hospital-acquired pneumonia, which is pneumonia contracted in the hospital. A newly designated health care–associated pneumonia (HCAP)

Disclosure Statement: The authors have nothing to disclose.
MEDEX Northwest PA Program, Department of Family Medicine, University of Washington, 4311 11th Avenue Northeast, Suite 200, Seattle, WA 98105, USA
* Corresponding author.
E-mail address: Sls47@uw.edu

is defined as pneumonia that is acquired in the community by people who have been exposed to pathogens from a hospital.[7] For example, patients in a long-term care facility or a rehabilitation center. Unfortunately, HCAP guidelines recommend triple or quadruple antibiotic therapy and may lead to overusage of antibiotics in the outpatient setting.[7] This article does not address HCAP; however, most of these patients without complications or further comorbidities can be managed in a manner similar to that discussed in this article by using the current CAP guidelines.[3,7]

EPIDEMIOLOGY OF COMMUNITY-ACQUIRED PNEUMONIA

Many providers will encounter patients with CAP over the course of their career. CAP is the number 1 cause of infection and "sometimes the forgotten killer" throughout the world, at any age.[1,2] In the United States, it is 1 of the 10 leading causes of death and is a costly burden on the health care system. Current estimates of death from CAP are approximately 137 deaths per day.[1] However, that number may be underestimated, as many patients die from other complications, such as sepsis, cancer, and Alzheimer disease, and CAP is not the primary diagnosis code on the death certificate.[1] It is better to have not had CAP in your lifetime, as a recent study showed that patients who have not had CAP have less long-term health sequelae compared with those patients who have had CAP, regardless of age.[8]

ETIOLOGY

It is important to understand the most likely causes of CAP so as to guide the management and treatment of the infection. The most likely etiologic pathogens that cause CAP differ between children and adults. Discovering the etiologic pathogen in children can be challenging.[5] In 2011, guidelines by the Pediatric Infectious Diseases Society and the Infectious Diseases Society of America were published for the management of CAP in infants and children older than 3 months.[5] These guidelines mention the difficulty in determining the exact pathogen causing CAP, which usually is a combination of both viral and bacterial pathogens[5] (Table 1).

The guidelines state, however, that children younger than 2 years present more commonly with viral pneumonia associated with the respiratory syncytial virus (RSV).[5] However, children older than 10 years present with bacterial forms of CAP.[5] With regard to "atypical forms of CAP," in older children, *Mycoplasma pneumoniae* is identified in approximately 25% of those children, whereas infants present with *Chlamydophila pneumoniae*.[5] *Legionella* is rare in children.[5] It is rare to find a fungal cause for pneumonia in both adults and children. Those patients at highest risk for tuberculosis (TB) should be screened based on risk factors and suspicion of TB.

Table 1
Pathogens in community-acquired pneumonia: pediatric outpatient setting

1–3 Mo of Age	>3 Mo Old
Respiratory syncytial virus, influenza, rhinovirus, parainfluenza virus, adenovirus, human metapneumovirus	Same viruses as 1–3 mo
Bordetella pertussis	*Streptococcus pneumoniae*
S pneumoniae	*Haemophilus influenzae*
Staphylococcus aureus (rare)	*Mycoplasma pneumoniae*

Data from Refs.[5,11,14]

For an adult patient with CAP, think of "typical versus atypical" bacterial pathogens[1] (Tables 2 and 3).

In adults, approximately 50% of the cases present with the typical bacterial pathogen of *Streptococcus pneumoniae* (also known as pneumococcus) and the most common atypical bacterial pathogens, which manifest in up to 30% of CAP, are *Mycoplasma pneumoniae* or *Chlamydophila pneumoniae*[3] (see Table 2). A third atypical pathogen implicated in more severe cases of CAP is *Legionella*.[3] The last 2 causative bacterial pathogens, *Haemophilus influenzae* and *Moraxella catarrhalis*, are found more often in the geriatric population or in patients with underlying lung diseases and/or chronic obstructive pulmonary disease (COPD).[1,3] The most common respiratory viral etiology is influenza. Influenza places patients at risk for developing a secondary bacterial CAP infection, in which *Staphylococcus aureus* is frequently identified. All of this is important to keep in mind when deciding on treatment therapies, which are discussed later.

PATHOPHYSIOLOGY

Pneumonia develops from an overproduction of microbial pathogens in the alveoli.[9] If an individual's immune defense mechanisms are unable to fight the bacterial, viral, fungal, or parasitic invasion, the various microbes overgrow and produce an infection in the lung tissue.[9] There are 3 mechanisms described as causes for developing pneumonia. The most common means of transmission is through small aspirations from the oropharynx into the lung. A second cause is from infected respiratory droplets that are inhaled into the lower respiratory tract; rarely does pneumonia develop from vascular sources or pleural spaces.[9]

CLINICAL MANIFESTATIONS

Taking a careful and complete history of the patient is important in making the diagnosis of CAP. Recent exposure and travel history may be helpful in identifying probable pathogens. The clinical manifestations of CAP in children and adults can be varied, depending on age. The most common presenting signs and symptoms of cough, with or without fever, are nonspecific, but suggestive of pneumonia.[5] Typical signs and symptoms of *S pneumoniae* present with high fever, productive cough, and abnormal lung findings in one lobe, whereas atypical CAP pathogens, such as *M pneumoniae*, present with a low-grade fever, nonproductive cough, and nonspecific abnormal lung sounds. In children, the younger the child, the more difficult CAP can be to diagnose, as infants may present with fussiness and poor feeding. After the

Table 2 "Typical versus atypical" pathogens in community acquired pneumonia: adult outpatient setting	
Typical	**Atypical**
Streptococcus pneumoniae	Mycoplasma pneumoniae
Haemophilus influenzae	Chlamydophila pneumoniae
Moraxella catarrhalis	Respiratory viruses
	Legionella pneumophila

Adapted from Solomon CG, Wunderink RG, Waterer GW. Community-acquired pneumonia. N Engl J Med 2014;370(6):543–51; and Antimicrobial therapy. Sanford Guide Web Edition Web site. Available at: http://webedition.sanfordguide.com/sanford-guide-online. Accessed June 28, 2016.

Table 3		
CURB65: criteria for admission to the hospital for CAP		
C	Confusion	1 point
U	Blood urea nitrogen >19 mg/dL	1 point
R	Respiratory rate >30 min	1 point
B	Blood pressure <90/60	1 point
65	≥65 y	1 point

Scoring: greater than 1 point = hospital admission.
From Mandell LA, Wunderink RG, Anzueto A, et al. Infectious Diseases Society of America/American Thoracic Society consensus guidelines on the management of community acquired pneumonia in adults. Clin Infect Dis 2007;44:S27–72.

age of 10, children and adults present more classically with a cough, fever, and, on auscultation, decreased breath sounds or crackles or rhonchi in one particular area of the lung.[5] If a patient is dehydrated, auscultation of the breath sounds may be more difficult and the abnormal breath sounds may not be as pronounced until the patient is rehydrated. Any patient in respiratory distress requires hospitalization.[5] In neonates or infants who present with grunting, intercostal rib retractions, increased respiratory rates (>50–70 breaths per minute), or a pulse oximetry at or below 90% to 92% on room air, will require inpatient management and treatment.[5] Older children and adults who present with vomiting, dehydration, increased respirations, and a low pulse oximetry, at or below 90% to 92% on room air, should be considered for admission.[5,9] Pneumonia may present more subtly, with abdominal pain, due to referred pain from the lower lung lobes or stiffness in the neck from referred pain in the upper lobes.[9]

DIAGNOSTIC TESTING

Diagnostic and laboratory testing guidelines differ between children and adults with CAP. Pediatric patients presenting with uncomplicated CAP do not require a chest radiograph in the outpatient setting.[5] A chest radiograph should be ordered if a patient is not responding to treatment (fever persisting or clinical deterioration) within 48 to 72 hours of the diagnosis. Routine follow-up chest radiographs are also not recommended in the pediatric population.[5] However, if a patient has a reoccurring pneumonia in the same lung area, a chest radiograph should be ordered and a follow-up chest radiograph is needed at 4 to 6 weeks. Any pediatric patient who is admitted to the hospital should have a posteroanterior (PA) and lateral chest radiograph to guide in the management and treatment of the CAP.[3,10]

Adults should have a chest radiograph in cases in which CAP is suspected, even in the outpatient setting.[3] With regard to laboratory testing, in the outpatient setting, testing should be used to guide the choice of antibiotic or antiviral medication. Rapid influenza testing is available and can aid in the treatment with an antiviral medication and prevent overuse of antibiotics, unless a secondary bacterial infection is suspected.[5,9] Other laboratory testing, such as sputum cultures, blood cultures, or specific urinary antigen testing, should be reserved for hospitalized patients. A complete blood count (CBC) again should be ordered in a hospital setting but is not necessary in an uncomplicated outpatient setting. Other serologic tests, such as an erythrocyte sedimentation rate or C-reactive protein are acute-phase reactant tests and may be ordered in a hospital setting. Both the CBC and acute-phase reactant laboratory tests may help in determining if a pediatric patient is responding to medications and therapies and guide in decision making.[3] In the adult patients with CAP, monitoring of the CBC and acute-phase reactant is not mentioned; however, this could apply to an adult patient, depending on the severity of the infection.

MANAGEMENT AND TREATMENT

Most pediatric patients with CAP can be managed in the outpatient setting with close follow-up.[3,5] Box 1 describes the associated risk factors that predispose and increase the susceptibility to CAP in the pediatric patient.[11–13]

Criteria for hospitalization in children is chosen in infants and children with an increased respiratory rate of greater than 50 to 70 breaths per minute, pulse oximetry below 90% to 92% on room air, and vomiting with ensuing dehydration, comorbid conditions (eg, cardiovascular or pulmonary diseases), and failure to improve on outpatient therapy for 48 to 72 hours.[5] Neonates require hospitalization, as the likely pathogens are the same as in neonatal sepsis and intravenous antibiotics are imperative.[5] Encouraging fluids, rest, and antipyretics, if needed to decrease fever, is part of the initial plan for treatment of CAP. As mentioned earlier, infants and children usually present with viral pathogens as the cause, so an antiviral agent may be the best choice.[4,5,14] High-dosage amoxicillin for 7 days is preferred for infants and preschool children when a bacterial pathogen is suspected and the child has been appropriately immunized. In immunized children who are suspected of an atypical pneumonia, a macrolide antibiotic should be used.[4,5,14] (Box 2).

Deciding when to hospitalize an adult patient guides management and treatment options. One tool, developed by the British Thoracic Society in 1987, is frequently used to determine whether an adult patient can be managed in the outpatient setting or needs inpatient treatment and is used as a severity risk assessment tool. This is called CURB65, which stands for level of confusion, urea level, respiratory rate, blood pressure, and age greater than or equal to 65[15–17] (see Box 1).

Scoring 1 to 2 points, the health care provider should consider hospitalization or close monitoring in the outpatient setting. Above 2 points in any criterion requires that the patient be admitted to the hospital. The higher the score, the higher the mortality.[3,16,17] The Pneumonia Severity Index is a more comprehensive tool that looks at 20 different patient variables and predicts mortality more accurately; however, due to its complexity, it is not as widely used as the CURB65.[16]

Box 1
Risk factors that influence increased risk for community-acquired pneumonia in children

Neonates born at age 24 to 28 weeks

Lower socioeconomic status

Second-hand smoke

No childhood immunizations

Underlying cardiac disease

Underlying pulmonary disease

Immunodeficiency

Underlying neuromuscular disease

Data from Refs.[11–13]

> **Box 2**
> **Treatment for CAP in an infant or child**
>
> Amoxicillin 90–100 mg/kg/day q 12 hours for 7 days OR
>
> Azithromycin 10 mg/kg po day one (max of 500 mg), then 5 mg/kg (max of 250 mg) po for 4 days
>
> *Abbreviations:* Po, by mouth; q, every.
>   *Data from* Ananda-Rajah MR, Charles PG, Melvani S, et al. Comparing the pneumonia severity index with CURB-65 in patients admitted with community acquired pneumonia. Scand J Infect Dis. 2008:40(4):293–300.

When choosing an antibiotic for a suspected bacterial cause of CAP, the importance of knowing the resistance rates in the area are imperative.[3,14] Keeping in mind the resistance patterns, if greater than 25% resistance of S pneumoniae is reported, then alternative treatment options should be considered[14] (Fig. 1).

For the first-line treatment of an uncomplicated, no comorbidity CAP in an adult, it is best to start with a macrolide antibiotic (azithromycin or clarithromycin) and use doxycycline or an oral cephalosporin as an alternative treatment[14] (see Fig. 1). For those patients with a comorbidity (Box 3), start with levofloxacin (see Fig. 1).[14]

Fortunately, the fluoroquinolone class of antibiotics still has benefits that outweigh the risks and are still indicated in the treatment of CAP even though they have developed increased resistance, and the potential side effects have brought additional precautions from the Food and Drug Administration when choosing from this class of antibiotics for less severe infections.[18,19]

If a patient is positive for influenza A or B, antibiotics can be discontinued after 24 hours, unless a secondary bacterial infection is suspected.[14] As mentioned previously, if the patient is positive for influenza type A or B, an antiviral agent, which reduces the viruses ability to replicate, should be initiated. Currently, zanamivir and oseltamivir should generally be prescribed within the first 48 hours of symptoms to be most effective.[14] Both of these should reduce the number of days with the illness and also decrease the severity of the symptoms associated with influenza. Resistance also has occurred to influenza with older antiviral agents, such as amantadine and rimantadine, and, therefore, these agents are used less frequently.[3]

Once an antibiotic and or an antiviral medication is initiated, close follow-up and individualized care are critical in determining if the treatment is effective. Other medications may be considered in addition to the antibiotic or antiviral. For example, corticosteroids, such as prednisone, should be reserved for those patients with asthma, COPD, or other underlying lung disorders that may warrant more aggressive treatment of the additional inflammation caused by the underlying lung disease.[20] In otherwise healthy individuals, corticosteroids are not recommended.[3] Other medications to improve cough, such as guaifenesin, a mucolytic, is sometimes suggested clinically but has not been proven to be better than placebo in clinical trials. Cough suppressants are usually discouraged, as it is best to cough up the mucous rather than suppress the cough.[21]

Close follow-up care is important to ensure that the patient is recovering. In the outpatient setting, having a patient return in 2 days determines if you have chosen the best treatment plan. In 2 days, if not improving or if symptoms have worsened, then a chest radiograph is warranted and adding or changing medications may be warranted.[3] If the patient is improving steadily, further follow-up in 2 to 4 weeks is beneficial to determine total resolution of the pneumonia.

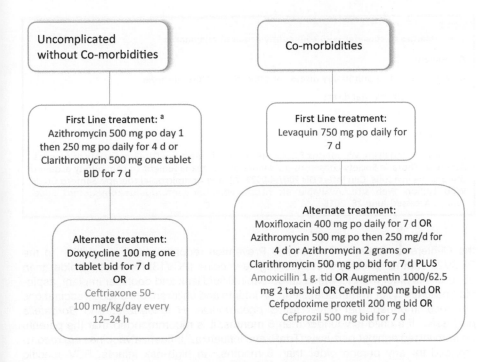

Fig. 1. Treatment for CAP in an adult outpatient setting. Bid, twice a day; tid, 3 times a day. [a] If >30% resistance to *s. pneumoniae* go to alternate therapy. If on antibiotics in the past 3 months then First line treatment PLUS Amoxicillin 1 g. tid OR Augmentin 1000/62.5mg 2 tablets bid OR Levaquin 750mg one tablet daily for 7 days. (*Data from* Mandell LA, Wunderink RG, Anzueto A, et al. Infectious Diseases Society of America/American Thoracic Society consensus guidelines on the management of community acquired pneumonia in adults. Clin Infect Dis. 2007;44:S27–S72; and Ananda-Rajah MR, Charles PG, Melvani S, et al. Comparing the pneumonia severity index with CURB-65 in patients admitted with community acquired pneumonia. Scand J Infect Dis. 2008:40(4):293-300.)

PREVENTION OF COMMUNITY-ACQUIRED PNEUMONIA AND OTHER CONSIDERATIONS

The best way to treat CAP is to prevent it in the first place. Currently, we have vaccines that are effective in preventing *S pneumoniae*, antibiotic-resistant *S pneumoniae*, and influenza A and B, the 2 most common etiologies of CAP from infancy to adulthood.[2,3,5] There are more than 90 identified types of *S pneumoniae*.[2] Thirty-six types of the most common and more aggressive forms have been recognized.[2] Two of these vaccines that contain 24 serotypes are recommended. For the prevention of CAP with *S pneumoniae*, in adults older than 65, in patients 19 years or older with chronic health conditions, such as diabetes mellitus, smoking, liver disease, heart and lung diseases, and those that are immunocompromised, the pneumococcal polysaccharide vaccine (PPSV23) has been recommended. More recently,

Box 3
Comorbidities to consider with community-acquired pneumonia

Alcoholism

Chronic obstructive pulmonary disease or other chronic lung disorder

Chronic heart/liver/renal disease

Diabetes mellitus

Malignancy or other immunodeficiencies

Data from Mandell LA, Wunderink RG, Anzueto A, et al. Infectious Diseases Society of America/ American Thoracic Society consensus guidelines on the management of community acquired pneumonia in adults. Clin Infect Dis 2007;44:S27–72; and Antimicrobial therapy. Sanford Guide Web Edition Web site. Available at: http://webedition.sanfordguide.com/sanford-guide-online. Accessed June 28, 2016.

the Centers for Disease Control and Prevention recommended in addition to the PPSV23 another pneumococcal conjugate vaccine (PCV13) for patients older than 65, patients older than 19 with a cerebrospinal fluid leak and cochlear implant, asplenia, malignancy, or immunodeficient.[2] In infants and children, childhood vaccinations are recommended that cover for *S pneumoniae, H influenzae*, and *Bordetella pertussis*.[5] If a child is younger than 6 months, it is recommended that the parents be immunized against pertussis (TdaP) and influenza.[5] Influenza vaccines are recommended for any person older than 6 months.[2] In high-risk infants, RSV-specific monoclonal antibody is suggested to prevent RSV pneumonia, the most common form of CAP, in that age group.[2] Other considerations for prevention include smoking cessation, as this should always be encouraged at any age; as well as suggesting no second-hand smoke around other people at any age.[2]

SUMMARY

CAP, one of the most common and deadliest illnesses in the world, can be prevented, managed, and treated more effectively when following and recognizing the specific guidelines outlined for health care providers by the American and British Thoracic Societies and the Pediatric and Adult Infectious Diseases Societies of America. For the primary care clinician, focus should be on prevention first. Newer vaccines and recommendations for the prevention of *S pneumoniae*, resistant strains of *S pneumoniae*, and influenza A and B in adults and children should be followed. To further assist in treating the patient appropriately and also preventing further drug-resistant bacteria and viruses, antibiotics and antivirals should be prescribed according to the guidelines. Individualizing treatment of each patient with CAP and monitoring appropriately with close follow-up, should improve the overall outcomes and reduce mortality.

REFERENCES

1. Solomon CG, Wunderink RG, Waterer GW. Community-acquired pneumonia. N Engl J Med 2014;370(6):543–51.
2. Pneumonia. Centers for Disease Control and Prevention. Available at: http://www.cdc.gov/pneumonia. Accessed June 29, 2016.
3. Mandell LA, Wunderink RG, Anzueto A, et al. Infectious Diseases Society of America/American Thoracic Society consensus guidelines on the management of community acquired pneumonia in adults. Clin Infect Dis 2007;44:S27–72.

4. Harris M, Clark J, Coote N, et al. British Thoracic Society guidelines for the management of community acquired pneumonia in children: update 2011. Thorax 2011;66(Suppl 2):ii1–23.
5. Bradley JS, Byington CL, Shah SS, et al. The management of community-acquired pneumonia in infants and children older than 3 months of age: clinical practice guidelines by the Pediatric Infectious Diseases Society and the Infectious Diseases Society of America. Clin Infect Dis 2011;53(7):617–30.
6. Prina E, Ranzani O, Polverino E, et al. Risk factors associated with potentially antibiotic- resistant pathogens in community-acquired pneumonia. Ann Am Thorac Soc 2015;12(2):153–60.
7. Wunderink RG. Community-acquired pneumonia versus healthcare-associated pneumonia. The returning pendulum. Am J Respir Crit Care Med 2013;188(8):896–8.
8. Eurich DT, Marrie TJ, Minhas-Sandhu J, et al. Ten-year mortality after community-acquired pneumonia. A prospective cohort. Am J Respir Crit Care Med 2015;192(5):597–604.
9. Mandell LA, Wunderink RG. Pneumonia. In: Kasper D, Fauci A, Hauser S, et al, editors. Harrison's principles of internal medicine, 19e. New York: McGraw-Hill; 2015. p. 1–25.
10. Claessens YE, Debray MP, Tubach F, et al. Early chest computed tomography scan to assist diagnosis and guide treatment decision for suspected community-acquired pneumonia. Am J Respir Crit Care Med 2015;192(8):974–82.
11. Glezen P, Denny F. Epidemiology of acute lower respiratory disease in children. N Engl J Med 1973;288(10):498–505.
12. Green G, Carolin D. The depressant effect of cigarette smoke on the in vitro antibacterial activity of alveolar macrophages. N Engl J Med 1967;276(8):421–7.
13. Pelton S, Hammerschlag M. Overcoming current obstacles in the management of bacterial community-acquired pneumonia in ambulatory children. Clin Pediatr 2005;44(1):1–17.
14. Antimicrobial therapy. Sanford Guide Web Edition Web site. Available at: http://webedition.sanfordguide.com/sanford-guide-online. Accessed June 28, 2016.
15. Ananda-Rajah MR, Charles PG, Melvani S, et al. Comparing the pneumonia severity index with CURB-65 in patients admitted with community acquired pneumonia. Scand J Infect Dis 2008;40(4):293–300.
16. Aujesky D, Auble TE, Yearly DM, et al. Prospective comparison of three validated prediction rules for prognosis in community-acquired pneumonia. Am J Med 2005;118(4):384–92.
17. Jones BE, Jones J, Bewick T, et al. CURB-65 pneumonia severity assessment adapted for electronic decision support. Chest 2011;140(1):156–63.
18. Lai C, Lee K, Lin S, et al. Nemonoxacin (TG-873870) for treatment of community-acquired pneumonia. Expert Rev Anti Infect Ther 2014;12(4):401–17.
19. FDA Drug Safety Communication: FDA advises restricting fluoroquinolone antibiotic use for certain uncomplicated infections; warns about disabling side effects that can occur. Available at: http://www.fda.gov/Drugs/Drug Safety/ucm500 143.htm. Accessed June 28, 2016.
20. Wan YD, Sun TW, Liu ZQ, et al. Efficacy and safety of corticosteroids for community-acquired pneumonia: a systematic review and meta-analysis. Chest 2016;149(1):209–19.
21. Berlin CMJ, McCarver-May DG, Notterman DA, et al. Use of codeine- and dextromethorphan-containing cough remedies in children. Pediatrics 1997;99(6):918–20.

Skin and Soft Tissue Infections

Karen McMenemy, RPA-C, MS

KEYWORDS

- Skin and soft tissue infections • *Staphylococcus* • Abscess • *Streptococcus*
- Cellulitis • Polymicrobial cutaneous infection
- Acute bacterial skin and skin structure infection • Necrotizing skin infections

KEY POINTS

- Skin and soft tissue infections (SSTIs) are increasing in frequency, with drug-resistant organisms contributing to increased hospitalizations and health care utilization.
- Community-acquired and hospital-acquired methicillin-resistant *Staphylococcus aureus* (MRSA) is the major pathogen contributing to this increase and risk stratification for MRSA must be used to maximize treatment efficacy.
- *Staphylococcus* and *Streptococcus* species are predominant organisms of SSTIs, but anatomic location of infections and patient comorbid conditions may promote infection with less common organisms and require alteration of empirical therapy.
- Careful evaluation of patient clinical condition and situational epidemiology must be quickly and accurately performed to identify those in need of hospitalization, immediate intravenous antibiotics, and further workup or surgical intervention.
- Numerous antibiotics are available for use against SSTIs, and knowledge of their activity spectra, side effects, local resistance patterns against suspected pathogens, and administration cost must factor into the choice to provide the most efficacious therapy while minimizing side effects and unnecessary costs.

INTRODUCTION

When Alexander Fleming first concentrated the active substance he named penicillin in 1928, the world was a different place: soldiers in generations of wars were lost due to simple wounds that became infected and no treatment could provide relief. Children became deaf from ear infections, thousands had tragic complications from simple streptococcal throat infections, and women would die from childbirth due to infection. The 1945 Nobel Prize given to Chain, Fleming, and Florey for mass production of penicillin seemed like the promise of a new world in which simple bacterial infections could no longer threaten the populace. That dream lasted less than 100 years. Antibiotics

The author has nothing to disclose.
Department of Medicine, NYU-Lutheran Medical Center, 150-55th Street, Brooklyn, NY 11220, USA
E-mail address: ksmnypa@icloud.com

Physician Assist Clin 2 (2017) 165–176
http://dx.doi.org/10.1016/j.cpha.2016.12.014   **physicianassistant.theclinics.com**

were used, overused, and organisms became resistant. Still, innovation is not just for the microbe because the clinician continues to look toward antibiotics as the salvation from common infections in this young century.

Skin and soft tissue infections (SSTIs) cover a multitude of clinical presentations, ranging from mild, which require minimal intervention, to severe life-threatening infections, which demand immediate intravenous (IV) antibiotic administration and surgical intervention. Evaluation of infection severity and identification of the most likely causative organism promotes improved outcomes and decreases development of resistance in the microorganisms. New pharmacologic agents have increased options for treatment of these infections but must be used prudently to enhance long-term drug sensitivity and minimize health care costs.

Infections of the skin and soft tissue occur commonly and have been increasing rapidly over the last 30 years when methicillin-resistant *Staphylococcus aureus* (MRSA) began to emerge as a causative agent in hospital-acquired infections.[1,2] Before the 1990s, most MRSA was nosocomial[1] (termed health care-associated MRSA [HA-MRSA]) but resistance rates have continued to climb and community-acquired MRSA (CA-MRSA) has emerged as a widespread contributor to a 3-fold increase in emergency department visits[3,4] and hospitalizations.[5] Likewise, some isolates of enteric gram-negative bacteria have become more resistant and the increase of diabetes mellitus has placed a larger population at risk for these infections.[6] With initial treatment failure rates of SSTIs estimated to be between 15% and 30%, knowledge of local resistance patterns and stratification of risk for resistant strains becomes paramount to decrease both the indirect and direct costs to the medical system and society.[1,6]

To maximize efficacy of clinical empirical therapy, this article outlines evaluation and treatment of purulent infections, nonpurulent infections, polymicrobial and surgical infections, and the commonly used drugs recommended for these cases.

PURULENT SKIN INFECTIONS

The most common agent in purulent skin infections is *Staphylococcus aureus*.[6] Since the early 1990s, the emergence of MRSA has risen dramatically, with an increase of 50% since 2008.[4] Current rates of MRSA are approximately 30% to 50% of all staphylococcal isolates,[6,7] although true numbers are unclear because outpatient infections are not as frequently cultured and thus full-resistance patterns remain partially unknown.[1] Resistant strains of *Staphylococcus aureus* are frequently encountered in primary care situations and the clinician must have a high suspicion for MRSA to empirically cover in the high-risk patient, then deescalate therapy as cultures become available.[6]

Genetically, *Staphylococcus aureus* from nosocomial infections is distinctly different from CA-MRSA, and HA-MRSA strains are more often implicated in pneumonia or surgical site infections, rather than SSTIs.[2] However, in the last decade, increased prevalence of both strains has caused a more indistinct separation of infection spectra.[2] Overall, MRSA increases morbidity and relapse due to inadequate treatment or unrecognized resistance, and contributes to a higher incidence of mortality during the first year after diagnosis than in those patients without MRSA.[1]

Abscesses

Traditionally, purulent infections resulting in collections of pus in the dermis and deep tissues are associated with *Staphylococcus aureus*,[6] and remain the most common isolate in surgical infections and complicated skin infections.[8] In certain circumstances, however, abscesses can also be caused by gram-negative organisms, nontuberculous mycobacteria, and mixed bacterial isolates.[6,8,9]

Initial examinations of those with these infections may demonstrate symptoms of fever, skin erythema, edema, and frequently pustules or an area of localized fluctuance and induration.[2] Risk factors for purulent soft tissue infections include diabetes, extremes of age, institutionalized patients, and those participating in IV drug use.[1,10] Due to importance of drainage of abscesses in management of these infections, if it is unclear if an abscess exists, ultrasound can be used to quickly differentiate abscess versus cellulitis.[2,4,11]

If an abscess is demonstrated, incision and drainage are indicated,[2,6,11,12] and a culture is sent for identification and sensitivity.[3,12] After drainage is completed, current studies recommend against routine packing of wounds in straightforward, noncomplicated cases.[2,6,11,12] In cases of severe abscesses, a loop drain can be used in lieu of packing.[2] Although needle aspiration can be performed in cases in which it is difficult to access abscesses, or in situations in which the abscess cannot be immediately incised and drained, the rate of recurrence of these abscesses is increased by 50% compared with those drained by incision.[2]

Antibiotic administration is not routinely recommended in uncomplicated abscesses after successful incision and drainage.[2,11,12] However, if a patient has recurrent or severe disease, systemic toxicity, immunosuppression, or had inadequate drainage, antibiotics are recommended.[6,10,12] Children are usually prescribed linezolid or clindamycin because these drugs are also effective against Streptococcus and because doxycycline is not recommended for use in children younger than 8 years old.[12] For adults, oral regimens of 5 to 10 days with coverage for MRSA are recommended, using trimethoprim-sulfamethoxazole (TMP-SMX), clindamycin, linezolid, or doxycycline in cases of prior outpatient antibiotic failure, in those patients with history of MRSA, or those patients at high risk for resistant infection until cultures are available (Table 1).[1,2,6,10,12]

If patients are clinically unstable, have multiple comorbidities, immunosuppression, or are in extremes of age, IV antibiotics are recommended[1,4,6,10,11] and hospitalization should be considered. Blood cultures provide a low yield for isolation of causative organisms in uncomplicated SSTIs and are not routinely performed unless a patient is immunosuppressed, has malignancy, appears systemically toxic, or suffers from water immersion injuries, animal bites, or is a child younger than 1 year old.[4,11]

Recommended IV antibiotics for suspected MRSA include vancomycin, linezolid, tedizolid, daptomycin, tigecycline, telavancin, dalbavancin, oritavancin, and ceftaroline.[5,6,10,12] Vancomycin remains the first-line drug in treatment of these infections for most hospitalized patients[5,7,8,12] but close follow-up of cultures is recommended because it is inferior to penicillins for methicillin-sensitive Staphylococcus aureus (MSSA).[5,6] Linezolid, clindamycin, and vancomycin remain the most used agents for MRSA and MSSA in cases of typo I hypersensitivity reactions to beta-lactams.[6] Rifampin can be used in combination for severe MRSA infections but isolates form resistance to it quickly and it is not to be used as monotherapy (Table 2).[12]

Additionally, infections in areas at high risk for polymicrobial and gram-negative infections, such as those near genitals, axilla, or abdomen, may be covered by additional antibiotics, such as piperacillin-tazobactam, cefepime, or meropenem, providing gram-negative coverage until cultures are available.[2,3] Treatment courses for hospitalized patients are 7 to 14 days for soft tissue infections.[12] However, they may be extended to 4 to 5 weeks in cases of suspected osteomyelitis or concurrent endocarditis, and 3 to 4 weeks for penetrating hand wounds, synovitis,

Table 1
Oral treatment of *Staphylococcus aureus*

Drug Name	Maximum Adult Dosage	Notable Additional Microbial Coverage	Precautions
TMP-SMX	1 double-strength tablet twice daily	Variable coverage aerobic gram-negative rods	Hyperkalemia with chronic renal insufficiency
Clindamycin	450 mg 4 times daily	Anaerobes, *Streptococcus*	Increased risk *Clostridium difficile* colitis; variable resistance MRSA
Cephalexin[a]	500 mg 4 times daily	*Streptococcus*	Eosinophilia
Dicloxacillin[a]	500 mg 4 times daily	*Streptococcus*	Fever, rash, rare hemorrhagic cystitis
Doxycycline	100 mg twice daily	Aerobic gram-negative rods; *Vibrio*	Contraindicated in children <8 y; photosensitivity
Linezolid	600 mg twice daily	*Enterococcus* including VRE, *Streptococcus*	Myelosuppression if taken >2 wk; can precipitate SSRI syndrome; lactic acidosis
Tedizolid	200 mg once daily	*Enterococcus* including VRE, *Streptococcus*	Thrombocytopenia less severe than linezolid

Abbreviation: VRE, vancomycin-resistant enterococcus.
[a] Drug for methicillin-sensitive strains only.
Data from Refs.[2,3,5,11]

or polymyositis.[3,6] Antibiotics should be deescalated per cultures, and transition to oral agents and discharge home may be feasible in patients with clinical improvement, if a suitable oral agent is available, and if the patient is able to tolerate outpatient management.[2,4]

Recurrent Abscesses

If patients have recurrent abscesses, defined as 2 or more SSTIs at different sites over a 6-month period, especially those beginning in childhood, evaluation must take place for genetic defects, such as chronic granulomatous disease, and for chronic diseases, such as hidradenitis suppurativa.[3,13] If these conditions are found, initial abscess drainage and bacterial cultures are to be treated with appropriate antibiotics, and long-term management with fastidious hygiene measures and antibiotic prophylaxis can be used.[3,13]

Although clear causative relationship between MRSA colonization and a new-onset SSTI is debatable,[2] clear evidence does exist to attempt decolonization if maximization of hygiene and control of predisposing factors fails.[2,3,10,12] The most common areas of chronic colonization include the nares, axillae, skin folds, and fingernails.[2] Viable cultures of MRSA can be found in household fomites, including razors, bathroom surfaces, and personal care items.[2,12] Immediate family members in the same household can be decolonized as well if infection becomes present in multiple members of the same family.[2,3,10,12] Nasal decolonization with mupirocin twice daily for 5 days, and skin decolonization with dilute bleach baths or chlorhexidine washes for 5 to 14 days is recommended.[2,3,10,12]

Table 2
Intravenous treatment of *Staphylococcus aureus*

Drug	Maximum Adult Dosage	Notable Additional Microbial Coverage	Precautions
Cefazolin[a]	2 grams every 8 h	*Streptococcus*	Local phlebitis, hypersensitivity
Ceftolozane	600 mg twice daily	*Streptococcus*, aerobic gram-negative rods	Poor anaerobic coverage; does not treat *Enterococcus* sp
Clindamycin	600 mg every 8 h	Anaerobes, *Streptococcus*	Increases risk of *Clostridium difficile* colitis; variable inducible resistance against MRSA
Dalbavancin	1000 mg × 1 dose, then 500 mg × 1 dose	*Streptococcus*	Red person syndrome; elevations of ALT, not approved for use in children
Daptomycin	4 mg per kilogram once daily	*Enterococcus* including VRE, *Streptococcus*	Delayed eosinophilic pneumonia, myopathy, not for concomitant use with statins
Linezolid	600 mg twice daily	*Enterococcus* including VRE, *Streptococcus*	Myelosuppression if taken greater than 2 wk, can precipitate SSRI syndrome, lactic acidosis
Nafcillin[a]	2 g every 4 h	*Streptococcus*	Adjust dose in renal and hepatic dysfunction
Oritavancin	1200 mg 1 time dose	*Enterococcus, Streptococcus*	Nausea, vomiting, diarrhea
Quinupristin-dalfopristin	7.5 mg per kilogram twice daily	*Enterococcus* including VRE, *Streptococcus*	Severe myalgias; requires central line
Tedizolid	200 mg once daily	*Enterococcus* including VRE, *Streptococcus*	Less thrombocytopenia than linezolid
Telavancin	10 mg per kilogram once daily	*Enterococcus, Streptococcus*	Nephrotoxic; QT prolongation
Tigecycline	100 mg once, then 50 mg every 12 h	*Streptococcus*, aerobic gram-negative rods	Black box warning: increased all-cause mortality; recommended use in situations in which alternative treatments not suitable
Vancomycin	30 mg per kilogram per day, divided into 2 doses	*Streptococcus*	Nephrotoxic; ototoxic, red person syndrome; slow bactericidal; variable tissue penetration; requires therapeutic drug monitoring

Abbreviations: ALT, alanine aminotransferase; VRE, vancomycin-resistant *Enterococcus*.
[a] Drug for methicillin-sensitive strains only.
Data from Refs.[3,5,8,12]

NONPURULENT SKIN INFECTIONS

Cellulitis and erysipelas, a diffuse infection with spreading edema, erythema, fever, malaise, and induration without abscess formation,[4,5] is most frequently caused by beta-hemolytic *Streptococcus*. Although 70% to 90% of cellulitis is due to *Streptococcal* species,[11] *Staphylococcus aureus*, *Enterococcus* species, and gram-negative organisms such as *Escherichia coli*, *Klebsiella* species, *Enterobacter* species, and *Pseudomonas aeruginosa* are also implicated, especially in lower extremity wounds.[6] Severe cellulitic infections can demonstrate petechiae, ecchymosis, hemorrhagic bullae, and peau d'orange dimpling[14]; whereas in mild cases it is often confused with stasis dermatitis, eczema, or other dermatologic conditions, and diagnosis can often be delayed.[3,4,14]

The risk factors for cellulitis are the extremes of age, obesity, diabetes, prior cellulitis, venous insufficiency, peripheral vascular disease, trauma, insect or animal bites, ulceration, lymphedema, and dermatologic conditions such as eczema, dermatitis, and onychomycosis.[3,4,14] In 30% to 80% of cases, a noticeable portal of entry is identified,[14] and inspection of interdigital toe spaces should be evaluated for possible infection and fissuring to reduce recurrence after treatment.[14,15] Recurrence of cellulitis is most commonly seen in lower extremities and has been noted to be between 10% to 20% within the subsequent 3 years,[14] with the tibial area the site of highest risk.[3] High suspicion for reoccurrence and modification of risk factors is, therefore, crucial in long-term management of cellulitis.[14]

Once diagnosis is suspected and appropriate treatment is begun, 24 to 48 hours of initial worsening of erythema and inflammation may occur in affected areas due to release of enzymes due to pathogen destruction, and must be differentiated from treatment failure.[6,14] Evaluation of temperature curve, trending of white blood cell count, and demarcation of erythema margin can be used to help differentiate the 2 outcomes. If after 48 to 72 hours no improvement is seen, it is crucial to reassess wounds, with a new culture if possible, and evaluate for potential abscess.[2] Treatment is recommended to be 7 to 10 days but must be tailored to patient response.[2,14]

Blood cultures are rarely positive in cases of lower limb cellulitis but should be collected in the systemically ill or immunocompromised patient.[3,4,14] Hospitalization is recommended if the patient has failed outpatient oral therapy, has a poor vascular system, concurrent lymphedema, or appears septic.[3,8,14] Superficial cultures of wounds are of limited use, with high yield of mixed multiple skin flora. Empirical therapy is better guided by using knowledge of potential pathogenic organisms in the affected anatomic area and understanding local bacterial sensitivity patterns.[16] These cultures may be used, however, when a patient appears toxic and an immediate Gram stain may guide clinical decisions.[8,16] Deep tissue culture or biopsy have more predictive value for treatment success but bacterial load is lower, resulting in fewer positive cultures, especially if these cultures are obtained after empirical antibiotics are given during initial contact in the emergency room.[16]

In mild cases of cellulitis, topical mupirocin can be used in cases of localized impetigo,[3] with systemic treatment if multiple areas are involved or if patient appears ill.[2] In most situations in which systemic antibiotic therapy is warranted, the recommended first-line of treatment is with beta-lactam antibiotics such as amoxicillin or amoxicillin-clavulanate, cephalexin, or dicloxacillin,[6] with dual coverage for MRSA if IV drug use is suspected, the patient has a penetrating trauma, or if the patient is known to be colonized with MRSA. The choice between oral versus IV antibiotics depends on patient comorbidities, severity of infection, and patient medication allergies.[3,11]

In the previously discussed situations, doxycycline or TMP-SMX can be added to the beta-lactam antibiotic, or linezolid or clindamycin can be used as a single agent to cover both *Streptococcus* and MRSA.[3,6,12] High rates of resistance to erythromycin have been seen in *Staphylococcus* and *Streptococcus* isolates, and it is, therefore, not recommended for cellulitis.[6] TMP-SMX, minocycline, and doxycycline have high clinical failure rates for *Streptococcus* and should not be used in cases in which it is the suspected cause.[2,6,10–12]

In addition to antibiotics, a concurrent prednisone course with taper from 40 mg to 0 over 8 days can be administered to decrease both the duration of the initial episode and frequency of recurrence.[3] Nonsteroidal anti-inflammatory agents can be used in a similar manner, with dosing of ibuprofen at 400 mg orally every 6 hours for 5 days. Both adjuvants are thought to reduce tissue inflammation and decrease lymphatic damage, and thus improve outcome.[3,14] Choice of treatment must be tailored to patient comorbid conditions, and adjusted or omitted based on overall risk of masking symptoms in the critically ill patient.[14] In addition, minimizing predisposing conditions through such methods as promoting weight loss, limb elevation, tight glucose control, and massage of lymphedema fluid proximally can further decrease frequency and duration of cellulitis.[3,14]

NECROTIZING SOFT TISSUE INFECTIONS

Advanced age, immunosuppression, diabetes, and obesity increase risk of rapidly progressing necrotizing infections.[6,14] Although necrotizing infections are rare, affecting 500 to 1500 people in the United States per year, the sudden progression to septic shock and rapid destruction of tissue makes the exclusion of this diagnosis a priority in the systemically ill patient.[6,14]

Necrotizing soft tissue infections occur two-thirds of the time in the lower extremities,[3,15] and can be from trauma, bruise or strain,[3] extension from infections in the genital or anal regions in immunocompromised hosts,[14] or spread from water-associated wounds.[3,15] In typical necrotizing soft tissue infections, *Streptococcus* is the most isolated organism, followed by *Staphylococcus* and *Peptostreptococcus*.[3,15] Necrotizing infections spreading from genital or abdominal wounds, trauma, and perianal wounds are usually polymicrobial,[3,14] and should be covered with antibiotics covering gram-negative, anaerobic, and gram-positive organisms.[3]

The hallmark of necrotizing infections is pain disproportionate to appearance of wound, wood-hard induration, and red tract formation, as well as rapid progression of infection through dermis, subcutaneous tissue, and muscle with delineation along fascial planes.[3,6] Patients may have skin ecchymosis, bullae, and display toxic effects, leading to septic shock if not treated appropriately.[3,6] Computed tomography (CT) can be used to evaluate necrotizing fasciitis but if high likelihood of necrotizing infection exists, appropriate antibiotics and immediate surgical debridement is warranted without delay for imaging. Surgical consultation for wide excision of affected tissues and collection of surgical cultures is performed on an emergent basis.[3,6] In addition, patients are returned to the operating room within 24 to 36 hours for second evaluation and further debridement as needed.[3]

Initial antibiotic treatment of suspected necrotizing infections is based on anatomic location and the suspected pathogen involved.[1,3,15] Clindamycin is used to inhibit toxin production and control inflammation in all infections with suspected *Clostridium* or *Streptococcus* as the predominant pathogen, and is used in combination with penicillin.[6] If the anatomic area is at risk for mixed infection, broadened coverage for gram-negative and anaerobic organisms is used.[3] In Fournier gangrene, a specific type of necrotizing fasciitis of the genital area, predominately in middle-age men, the causative organisms most often implicated are *Pseudomonas* and *Staphylococcus*, and antibiotic choice typically includes vancomycin plus piperacillin-tazobactam or vancomycin plus a carbapenem (eg, meropenem).[3] If infection began secondary to trauma in water or in those patients in daily contact with seafood processing, *Aeromonas* and *Vibrio* are covered with addition of ciprofloxacin or doxycycline, respectively.[3,6,14]

PERIORBITAL AND ORBITAL CELLULITIS

Periorbital or preseptal cellulitis is usually nonpurulent, affecting the eyelid only, and is usually associated with local trauma or an insect bite.[17,18] Although initial IV antibiotics are recommended, uncomplicated cases of preseptal cellulitis can be treated with 1 to 2 weeks of antibiotics, with transition to oral antibiotics to finish the course.[6,17,18] It is recommended to continue treatment until all edema and erythema have completely resolved.[6]

Orbital or postseptal cellulitis is typically an extension of acute sinusitis and has a much higher risk for complications.[17,18] Because clinical symptoms of ptosis, marked edema of eyelid, and erythema can exist in both orbital and periorbital cellulitis, a high index of suspicion must exist to rule out orbital cellulitis or fluid collection.[17] Although occurring in only 15% of cases, orbital abscess can progress rapidly, with possibility of proptosis, visual loss, meningitis, or death if not treated appropriately.[18] Because small children can be difficult to assess for symptoms of diplopia or visual changes, CT scanning for evaluation of fluid collection and ophthalmology, as well as consult with an ear, nose, and throat specialist, should not be delayed. If a fluid collection is found, immediate surgical drainage should commence.[17,18]

The most common causative agent of periorbital and orbital cellulitis was traditionally *Hemophilus influenzae*; however, with routine vaccination against *H influenzae* in children, currently the most commonly implicated organisms are *Streptococcus*, *Staphylococcus*, *Peptostreptococcus*, *Bacteroides*, and *Fusarium* species.[17,18] Typical antibiotic regimens include a cephalosporin (eg, ceftriaxone or cefepime) plus vancomycin, or ampicillin-sulbactam plus vancomycin.[17,18] Treatment courses are tailored to response, can last for more than 2 to 3 weeks in cases of complicated orbital cellulitis, and should not conclude until all edema and erythema have completely resolved.[6]

MANAGEMENT OF SKIN AND SOFT TISSUE INFECTIONS IN THE NEUTROPENIC OR IMMUNOCOMPROMISED PATIENT

Aggressive treatment of the neutropenic or severely immunocompromised patient with an SSTI is paramount because they are at higher risk for polymicrobial infection, myonecrosis, necrotizing infections, and sepsis.[3,6] In addition, states of lowered immunity provide an increased risk for reactivation of varicella and herpes simplex infections, which can manifest as local recurrence or dermatomal distribution, or become disseminated.[3] In addition to morbidity from these conditions, they cause skin breakdown, which increases risk for secondary infection.[3,6,16]

Due to neutropenia or impaired immunologic response, fever incidence may be decreased, formation of purulent collections delayed, and local skin reactions muted.[3] For these reasons, it is important to be aggressive to determine extent of infection, and to begin antibiotic and surgical management as soon as possible. Blood cultures and imaging studies should be ordered to rule out abscesses and determine extent of disease.[3,4,14] Biopsies of skin may be required if no drainable abscess exists to evaluate for bacterial organisms and rule out contributing fungal, parasitic, or viral causes.

Concurrent administration of granulocyte-stimulating factors to resolve neutropenia, and expert consultation is vital for optimal outcomes.[3]

Surgical and Mixed Flora Infections

Fever in the postoperative patient is usually not due to SSTIs within 48 hours of surgery unless gas gangrene is present or if the wound is secondary to traumatic injury.[3] *Clostridium* and *Streptococcus pyogenes* are most commonly implicated in these early infections but by 4 days postoperatively these infections peak in incidence.[3] Normal flora organisms specific to the surgical site are more often causative agents.[8] In all patients suspected of surgical site infection, draw blood cultures if the patient appears systemically ill,[8] drain all abscesses, remove suture material, and send deep wound cultures.[3,8]

If the surgical wound has only superficial infection, no systemic antibiotics are needed, unless the patient is ill appearing or unstable.[3] In cases of deeper infection or a toxic patient, antibiotics are warranted, with coverage for MRSA and enteric gram-negative rods, and with the addition of anaerobic and pseudomonal coverage in axillary, genital, gastrointestinal, and perineal infections. Typical regimens include vancomycin plus piperacillin-tazobactam or a carbapenem (eg, meropenem), or vancomycin plus cefepime and metronidazole.[3,8] A full course of therapy is determined by culture, with de-escalation of antibiotic coverage as appropriate.[8] Overall, these infections are most often caused by *Staphylococcus* and *Streptococcus*; however, gram-negative organisms such as *Escherichia coli*, *Pseudomonas aeruginosa*, and *Klebsiella* species, are increasing in incidence, and these organisms can be multidrug-resistant.[8] Statistically, worse overall outcome is expected in mixed infections.[8]

If localized tissue destruction is present, from suspected early gangrene, necrotic chronic decubitus, or diabetic foot ulcers, treatment includes early surgical debridement with collection of intraoperative cultures and initiation of broad-spectrum antibiotics to cover anaerobes, MRSA, *Pseudomonas aeruginosa*, and other enteric gram rods until Gram stain culture can provide more targeted antibiotic coverage.[3,6,19,20] This early intervention can contribute to future reduction of amputation events, and decrease hospitalization time due to early reduction of infection load and earlier identification of resistant organisms.[20] Once the patient is stabilized, additional operations may be attempted to ensure all areas of necrotic material are removed.[3] The use of hyperbaric oxygen has not been proven to add additional benefit to debridement and antibiotic use in either gas gangrene or in management of the infection of the diabetic foot (Table 3).[3,20]

Pharmacologic Treatment of Skin and Soft Tissue Infections

Once diagnosis of SSTI is reached, appropriate antibiotics are started based on the patient's clinical status, drug allergies, inpatient versus outpatient status, and suspected organism based on location and epidemiology of disease.[5,6,8,12] Currently, recommended drugs for SSTIs with common use include oral options of tetracyclines; TMP-SMX; linezolid, clindamycin, penicillins and cephalosporins; and IV agents of tigecycline, vancomycin, daptomycin, linezolid, tedizolid, clindamycin, quinupristin-dalfopristin, telavancin, dalbavancin, oritavancin, and ceftaroline.[6,10,12]

Effectiveness of penetration into affected tissue, side-effect profiles, treatment course cost, ease of administration, and local resistance patterns influence initial choice of antibiotic in SSTIs.[6,12] Although vancomycin remains the most commonly used first-line drug for broad gram-positive coverage, slow increases of minimum inhibitory concentrations in selected MRSA isolates,[6] nephrotoxicity, slow bactericidal activity, and the need for therapeutic drug monitoring has led to use of alternative

Table 3
Drugs for *Streptococcus* and polymicrobial infections

Streptococcal Agents	Drug	Maximum Adult Dosage	Notable Additional Microbial Coverage	Precautions
Topical	Mupirocin	Twice daily	*Staphylococcus aureus*, MRSA	Ineffective against *Enterococcus*
Oral	Amoxicillin-clavulanate	875 mg twice daily	*Staphylococcus*; variable aerobic gram-negative coverage, anaerobes	Diarrhea, adjust dose per renal function, hypersensitivity
	Cephalexin	250 mg 4 times daily	*Staphylococcus*	Not effective against MRSA; eosinophilia
	Clindamycin	400 mg 4 times daily	MRSA, anaerobes	Increases risk of *C difficile* colitis; variable inducible resistance to MRSA
	Dicloxacillin	250 mg 4 times daily	*Staphylococcus*	Not effective against MRSA; fever, rash, rare hemorrhagic cystitis
IV	Cefazolin	2 g every 8 h	*Staphylococcus*	Not effective against MRSA; local phlebitis, hypersensitivity
	Clindamycin	900 mg every 8 h	See above	See above
	Nafcillin	2 g every 4 h	*Staphylococcus*	Adjust dose in renal and hepatic dysfunction
Mixed Infections	Carbapenems	Variable per drug	*Staphylococcus*, anaerobic gram-negatives, including ESBL and carbapenemase producers, anaerobes	Seizures, possible cross-reactivity in penicillin allergy with positive skin test
	Cephalosporins generations 3 & 4	Variable per drug	Limited *Staphylococcus*, aerobic gram-negative rods, variable anaerobes per drug	Cross-reactivity in penicillin allergy; 3rd generation increase incidence of *C difficile* colitis
	Clindamycin	400 mg 4 times daily	See above	See above
	Fluoroquinolones	Variable per drug	Limited *Staphylococcus*, aerobic gram negative rods, pseudomonas	Neurotoxicity, optic neuritis, risk of tendon rupture, not for use in children <16 y old due to cartilage injury, exacerbates myasthenia gravis, QT prolongation, *C difficile* colitis
	Metronidazole	500 mg every 8 h	Anaerobes, specifically *C difficile*, flagellated parasites	Metallic taste, nausea, disulfiram reactions with alcohol use
	Ampicillin-sulbactam	3 g every 6 h	*Staphylococcus*, variable gram-negative rods, anaerobes	Phlebitis, anaphylaxis, neutropenia, eosinophilia
	Piperacillin-tazobactam	3.375 mg q 8 h	*Staphylococcus*, aerobic gram-negative rods, enhanced pseudomonal coverage, anaerobes	Nausea, diarrhea, headache, thrombocytopenia, especially in renal patients

Abbreviation: ESBL, extended spectrum beta-lactamase.
Data from Refs.[3,5,6,12]

drugs when MRSA is suspected or type I hypersensitivity reactions to beta-lactams exists.[5,8] Side effects of these medications, cost, and/or accessibility of the drugs have provided some challenges for widespread use and most vancomycin IV alternatives, with exception of clindamycin, are used as second-line to third-line treatments.[6]

For coverage of *Streptococcus* and MSSA, cephalosporins and penicillins should be used as first-line agents, and have benefit of coverage for some gram-negative organisms.[5,8] Clindamycin and linezolid have coverage for both *Staphylococcus* and *Streptococcus*, and come in both parenteral and oral forms, and thus facilitate transition to outpatient therapy. In addition, more recently released antibiotics such as dalbavancin and oritavancin possess a long half-life, require only 1 to 2 doses, and are, therefore, potential drugs for use in selected patients to minimize hospitalization costs.[1,5] As health care costs increase, a shift toward use of longer acting agents and outpatient treatments may increase use of these medications.[1]

SUMMARY

SSTIs are among the most commonly encountered infections seen in both inpatient and outpatient settings. Emerging resistance has made empirical therapy more challenging but with meticulous patient evaluation, identification of the most likely causative organism, knowledge of local resistance patterns, and laboratory follow-up, the clinician can provide targeted antibiotic therapy to minimize health care costs and maximize clinical outcomes for patients. Exponential treatment options since 1942 when penicillin was released have occurred but the organisms have likewise evolved. Clinician behavior must evolve to allow the antibiotics to be preserved for generations to come.

REFERENCES

1. Pollack CV Jr, Amin A, Ford WT Jr, et al. Acute bacterial skin and skin structure infections (ABBSI): Practice guidelines for management and care transitions in the emergency department and hospital. J Emerg Med 2015;48(4):508–19.

2. Mistry RD. Skin and soft tissue infections. Pediatr Clin North Am 2013;60(5): 1063–82.

3. Stevens DL, Bisno AL, Chambers HF, et al. Practice guidelines for the diagnosis and management of skin and soft tissue infections: 2014 update by the Infectious Diseases Society of America. Clin Infect Dis 2014;59(2):e10–52.

4. Phoenix G, Das S, Joshi M. Diagnosis and management of cellulitis. BMJ 2012; 345:e4955.

5. Tran MC, Naumovski S, Goldstein EJ. The times they are a-changin': new antibacterials for skin and skin structure infection. Am J Clin Dermatol 2015;16(3): 137–46.

6. Min AN, Cerceo EA, Deitelzweig SB, et al. Hospitalist perspective on the treatment of skin and soft tissue infections. Mayo Clin Proc 2014;89(10):1435–51.

7. Yue J, Dong BR, Yang M, et al. Linezolid versus vancomycin for skin and soft tissue infections. Cochrane Database Syst Rev 2016;(1):CD008056.

8. Barie PS, Wilson SE. Impact of evolving epidemiology on treatments for complicated skin and skin structure infections: the surgical perspective. J Am Coll Surg 2015;220(1):105–16.

9. Atkins BL, Gottlieb T. Skin and soft tissue infections caused by nontuberculous mycobacteria. Curr Opin Infect Dis 2014;27(2):137–45.

10. Bergstrom KG. Less may be more for MRSA: the latest on antibiotics, the utility of packing an abscess, and decolonization strategies. J Drugs Dermatol 2014; 13(1):89–92.
11. Fenster DB, Renny MH, Ng C, et al. Scratching the surface: a review of skin and soft tissue infections in children. Curr Opin Pediatr 2015;27(3):303–7.
12. Liu C, Bayer A, Cosgrove SE, et al. Clinical practice guidelines by the Infectious Diseases Society of America for the treatment of Methicillin-Resistant *Staphylococcus aureus* infections in adults and children. Clin Infect Dis 2011;52(3): e18–55.
13. Alhusayen R, Shear NH. Pharmacologic interventions for hidradenitis suppurativa: what does the evidence say? Am J Clin Dermatol 2012;13(5):283–91.
14. Hirschmann JV, Raugi GJ. Lower limb cellulitis and its mimics: part I lower limb cellulitis. J Am Acad Dermatol 2012;67(2):163.e1-12.
15. Anakwenze OA, Milby AH, Gans I, et al. Foot and ankle infections: diagnosis and management. J Am Acad Orthop Surg 2012;20:684–93.
16. Chakraborti C, Le C, Yanofsky A. Sensitivity of superficial cultures in lower extremity wounds. J Hosp Med 2010;5(7):415–20.
17. Rashed F, Cannon A, Heaton PA, et al. Diagnosis, management, and treatment of orbital and periorbital cellulitis in children. Emerg Nurse 2016;24(1):30–5.
18. Bedwell J, Bauman NM. Management of pediatric orbital cellulitis and abscess. Curr Opin Otolaryngol Head Neck Surg 2011;19(6):467–73.
19. Ramakant P, Verma AK, Misra R, et al. Changing microbiological profile of pathogenic bacteria in diabetic foot infections: time for a rethink on which empirical therapy to choose? Diabetologia 2011;54:58–64.
20. Peters EJ, Lipsky BA, Berendt AR, et al. A systematic review of the effectiveness of interventions in the management of infection in the diabetic foot. Diabetes Metab Rev 2012;24(supplement 1):S145–61.

Key Points Review of Meningitis

Susan Sweeney Stewart, PA-C, MPH, MMSc

KEYWORDS

- Bacterial meningitis • Viral meningitis • Meningitis treatment • Meningitis vaccines

KEY POINTS

- Hospitalization is usually required for appropriate management of suspected meningitis for rapid administration of intravenous antibiotics and antivirals, diagnostic testing, and pain management.
- Diagnosis of meningitis rests on the cerebrospinal fluid examination.
- Broad-spectrum antibiotics should be narrowed if bacterial cause found or stopped if viral, fungal, or mycobacterial cause found.

INTRODUCTION

When evaluating a patient for meningitis, it is best to prepare for the worst and hope for the best. Among lay people and patients' family members, the word meningitis can be very alarming. Certainly, *Neisseria meningitidis* is very serious with mortality between 9% and 73%, depending on serotype.[1] Alternatively, viral meningitis is usually self-limiting. Knowing epidemiologic risk factors and correlating patient symptoms and cerebrospinal fluid (CSF) findings with the various meningitis causes can help determine a differential diagnosis. Subsequently, the clinician will also know the appropriate management strategy. Some details of this are shared in this article. As a pretest, try answering the following questions:

1. What is the most common etiologic agent that causes meningitis in the United States?
2. What is the most common bacterium that causes meningitis in the United States?
3. What antibiotics should be initiated for suspected bacterial meningitis in the United States for adult patients with no past medical history?

Please check your answers at the end.

The author has nothing to disclose.
Atlanta ID Group, 275 Collier Road, Suite 450, Atlanta, GA 30309, USA
E-mail address: sjsweeney35@yahoo.com

Physician Assist Clin 2 (2017) 177–190
http://dx.doi.org/10.1016/j.cpha.2016.12.002   **physicianassistant.theclinics.com**

OVERVIEW AND EPIDEMIOLOGY

Meningitis is an inflammatory disease of the leptomeninges, the tissues surrounding the brain and spinal cord, and is defined by an abnormal number of white blood cells (WBCs) in the CSF. Most cases of meningitis in the United States are caused by a viral infection, but bacterial and fungal infections are also seen. According to reports from the Centers for Disease Control and Prevention (CDC), inpatient hospitalizations resulting from viral meningitis range from 25,000 to 50,000 each year, but the actual incidence may be as high as 75,000.[2] Several viruses produce aseptic (nonbacterial) meningitis, including enteroviruses, which are most common, followed by herpes simplex virus (HSV), varicella-zoster virus (VZV),[3,4] and then human immunodeficiency virus (HIV) and West Nile virus (WNV). According to the CDC, there were 4100 cases of bacterial meningitis, including 500 deaths, which occurred in the United States each year between 2003 and 2007.[5] Bacterial meningitis can be community-acquired or health care associated. The major causes of community-acquired bacterial meningitis in adults are *Streptococcus pneumoniae* (ie, Pneumococcus) with a prevalence rate of 61%, followed by *N meningitides* (ie, Meningococcus) (11%), *Haemophilus influenzae* (7%), *Listeria monocytogenes* (2%),[6] Group B streptococcus (in infants) (7%),[3] and tick-borne illnesses.[4] The major causes of health care–associated bacterial meningitis are staphylococci (including methicillin-resistant *Staphylococcus aureus*) and gram-negative bacilli, such as *Pseudomonas aeruginosa*. Meningitis can also be caused by various fungi, such as Cryptococcus, and can also be caused by *Mycobacterium tuberculosis*. Aseptic meningitis can be caused by malignancies, by autoimmune disorders, or can be medication induced. It is important to know the specific cause of meningitis because the treatment differs depending on the cause (Table 1).

CAUSE
Bacterial Meningitis

Streptococcus pneumoniae

The leading cause of bacterial meningitis in the United States is *S pneumoniae*. This bacterium is normally found in the respiratory tract of humans. Risk factors for *S pneumoniae* meningitis include immunosuppressive conditions, basilar skull fractures, and CSF leaks. If a contiguous or distant focus of infection is found (eg, sinusitis or brain abscess), consultation with an otorhinolaryngologist should be obtained. In a CDC study, there was a 59% decline in the rates of pneumococcal meningitis in children younger than 2 years of age after licensure of the heptavalent pneumococcal conjugate vaccine.[7] More recently, vaccination with PCV13 in France showed a decrease in the incidence of invasive pneumococcal disease (IPD) through 2012 in children up to the age of 5 but not in older children and adults.[8] Although among the immunosuppressed population IPD incidence decreased from 20 to 8/100,000-population year (*P*<.004) over the study period through 2014, no changes in mortality were observed. Penicillin resistance experienced a significant decline as well.[9]

Neisseria meningitidis

In young adults and teens, the bacterium *N meningitidis* causes meningococcal disease, which can be fatal if treatment is not initiated immediately. This bacterium is common and also lives naturally in the posterior nasopharynx. Human beings are the only place where meningococcal bacteria can live. At any one time, 10% to 25% of us carry the bacteria for weeks or months without ever knowing they are there.[10] For most of us, this is harmless because we have natural resistance. It is

Table 1
Characteristic features of common causes of bacterial meningitis by age and initial antibiotics

Age	Organism	Predisposing Condition	Initial Antibiotics
Neonates	Group B streptococcus, Escherichia coli, L monocytogenes, Klebsiella spp	Defects in cell-mediated immunity (immature immune system)	Ampicillin 100 mg/kg every 6 h PLUS cefotaxime 50 mg/kg every 6 h OR aminoglycoside (gentamicin 2.5 mg/kg every 8 h)
1–23 mo	S pneumoniae, N meningitides, Group B streptococcus, H influenzae, E coli	Defects in cell-mediated or humoral immunity	Vancomycin 15 mg/kg every 6–8 h PLUS Ceftriaxone 50 mg/kg every 12 h OR cefotaxime 150–300 mg/kg divided daily every 6–8 h
2–50 y	N meningitides, S pneumoniae	Usually none, rarely complement deficiency; all conditions that predispose to pneumococcal bacteremia, fracture of cribriform plate, cochlear implants, CSF otorrhea from basilar skull fracture, defects of the ear ossicle	Vancomycin 15 mg/kg every 6–12 h PLUS Ceftriaxone 2 g every 12 h or cefotaxime 2-3 g every 6–8 h
>50 y	S pneumoniae, N meningitides, L monocytogenes, gram-negative bacilli, S aureus, Coagulase-negative staphylococcus	Defects in immunity (HIV, transplant or chemotherapy patients), CSF leak, endocarditis, surgery, foreign body (especially ventricular drain)	Ceftriaxone 2 g every 12 h or cefotaxime 2-3 g every 6–8 h PLUS Ampicillin 2 g every 4 h PLUS Vancomycin 15–20 mg/kg every 12 h
Any age	S pneumoniae, H influenzae, gram-negative bacilli (including Pseudomonas), Anaerobic or microaerophilic streptococci, Bacteroides, S aureus	Sinusitis, otitis, CSF leak	ID consult recommended. Vancomycin PLUS Ceftazidime or Meropenem PLUS Metronidazole
Any age	S aureus, Coagulase-negative staphylococcus, gram-negative bacilli (including Pseudomonas) S pneumoniae	Penetrating head wound, neurosurgical procedure, shunt infection	ID consult recommended. Vancomycin plus Ceftazidime

Data from Greenlee JE. Merck Manual Professional Version. Overview of meningitis. Available at: http://www.merckmanuals.com/professional/neurologic-disorders/meningitis/overview-of-mening itis. Accessed September 23, 2016; and Tunkel AR, Hartman BJ, Kaplan SL, et al. Practice guidelines for the management of bacterial meningitis. Clin Infect Dis 2004;39:1267–84.

not known why these bacteria sometimes travel either via hematogenous or contiguous spread to the nervous system and cause meningitis. An antecedent upper respiratory infection may be a contributing factor.[11] Another proposed mechanism has been that physical damage to the epithelial cells lining the nose and throat permits easy passage of the bacteria into the bloodstream, causing invasive disease.[12] The bacteria are passed from person to person through prolonged close contact: coughing, sneezing, breathing each other's breath, or kissing someone who is carrying the bacteria. The bacteria are so fragile that they cannot survive for more than a few moments outside the human body. For this reason, they cannot be carried on things like cups, toys, furniture, or clothing. Having a weakened immune system also increases the risk for meningitis.

Other bacterial causes of meningitis include *H influenzae* type B (Hib) (although uncommon now since the introduction of the Hib vaccine), *L monocytogenes*, and Group B streptococcus. In addition, other bacterial causes that are frequently classified as "aseptic" given their CSF findings include *Treponema pallidum* (ie, syphilis) and vector-borne bacteria such as *Borrelia burgdorferi* (Lyme disease), *Rickettsia rickettsii* (Rocky Mountain spotted fever), Ehrlichia, and Anaplasma. Last, patients with a history of neurosurgical procedures (eg, CSF shunts) or trauma (eg, basilar skull fractures) are more likely to have health care–associated bacterial meningitis, which is usually caused by gram-negative bacilli or staphylococci.

Aseptic (Nonbacterial) Meningitis

Viruses

Enteroviruses In one prospective study in Finland, enteroviruses were the major causative agent (26%) followed by HSV-2 (17%) and VZV (8%).[4] Similarly, according to the CDC (especially in summer months), most viral meningitis cases are caused by enteroviruses.[13] Enteroviruses are a group of viruses that includes specific enteroviruses such as polioviruses, coxsackieviruses, and echoviruses. To determine viral cause, specimens such as CSF, stool or rectal swabs, blister fluid, throat swab, or blood can be tested to confirm cause. Enteroviral infection is suggested by the following: exanthemas, pericarditis, myocarditis, conjunctivitis, pleurodynia, herpangina, and hand, foot, and mouth disease. Enteroviruses are easily transmitted. An infected person may spread the viruses through close personal contact such as kissing, the air (through coughing or sneezing), contact with feces, or contact with contaminated objects and surfaces such as a doorknob and then touching your eyes, mouth, or nose. Generally, a person with hand, foot, and mouth disease is most contagious during the first week of illness. People can sometimes be contagious for days or weeks after symptoms go away. Some people, especially adults, may not develop any symptoms, but they can still spread the virus to others. For this reason, maintaining good hand hygiene is so important to minimize spreading the infection.

Herpes viruses Cases of herpetic meningitis are mainly described in immunocompetent patients, and HSV-2 is usually identified as the cause. HSV-2 meningitis is usually observed in the context of primary genital HSV-2 infection, but it can also be associated with recurrent genital herpes. It is also a classical cause of recurrent lymphocytic meningitis. Herpes viruses gain access to the central nervous system (CNS) by traveling in a retrograde fashion from peripheral nerve endings.[14] Antiviral therapy is most effective when started early. VZV is ubiquitous throughout the world. Initial infection with VZV results in chickenpox (varicella), which is typically seen in children aged 1 to 9 years. Chickenpox is seen less with the introduction of the Varivax vaccine. Recent data suggest that CNS complications caused by VZV reactivation are more common than previously thought.[15] Because these are treatable viruses, patients with suspected meningitis are usually given acyclovir upon presentation.

Other viruses that produce aseptic meningitis include HIV, WNV, mumps, lymphocytic choriomeningitis virus (airborne exposure to infected wild mice or pet hamsters), and cytomegalovirus[4,16] (Table 2).

Tuberculous

Tuberculosis (TB) meningitis (TBM) in the United States is a disease of young children with primary infection and patients with immunodeficiency seen with reactivation caused by aging, malnutrition, or disorders such as HIV and cancer. It is rare, with 100 to 150 cases occurring annually in the United States. Most patients have no known history of TB, but evidence of extrameningeal disease (pulmonary) can be found in about half of patients. The tuberculin skin test is positive in only about 50% of patients with TBM.[17] Duration of symptoms is usually subacute with onset of symptoms between 7 and 12 days of presentation, which is much longer than bacterial or viral meningitis.[3]

Fungal

Cryptococcosis Two varieties of Cryptococcus are recognized, variety *neoformans*, and variety *gattii*. *Cryptococcus neoformans* is found worldwide in association with soil contaminated with bird excreta. Serologic studies suggest that most individuals are exposed to the organism, starting after the first 2 years of life.[18] Cryptococcal meningitis is primarily a disease seen in persons with advanced HIV, although cases can occur in HIV-negative and nonimmunosuppressed patients as well. Duration of symptoms is also usually subacute with onset between 2 to 3 weeks of presentation.

Other fungal infections in the CSF that are even rarer include *Coccidioides immitis*, *Blastomyces dermatitidis*, and *Histoplasma capsulatum*.

Noninfectious

Meningitis can also be caused by cancers (eg, lymphoma), autoimmune disease such as lupus, multiple sclerosis, sarcoidosis, Guillain-Barré syndrome, certain drugs (eg,

Table 2
Common causes of viral meningitis

Viruses	Mechanism of Transmission	Seasonal Incidence
Enteroviruses	Fecal-oral spread (via contaminated food, in swimming pools)	Summer to early autumn, sometimes sporadic cases throughout year
Herpes simplex, usually virus type 2; may occur as an isolated instance or may recur	Sexual	None
VZV	Inhalation of respiratory droplets from or by contact with an infected person	None
WNV	Mosquito	Summer to early autumn
HIV usually associated with seroconversion	Contact with body fluids of infected person	None

Data from Greenlee JE. Merck Manual Professional Version. Overview of meningitis. 2015. Available at: http://www.merckmanuals.com/professional/neurologic-disorders/meningitis/over view-of-meningitis. Accessed September 23, 2016.

nonsteroidal anti-inflammatory drugs [NSAIDs]) or interestingly the combination of both autoimmune and NSAIDs.[19] Other drugs that are implicated include infliximab, carbamazepine, lamotrigine, antibiotics such as ciprofloxacin, penicillin, metronidazole, and trimethoprim-sulfamethoxazole. The underlying pathophysiology is thought to be due to a delayed hypersensitivity response to direct irritation of the meninges by the drug.[14]

HISTORY AND CLINICAL MANIFESTATIONS

Clues in the history include asking about past medical history of neurosurgical procedures, autoimmune disease, immunosuppressant use, TB diagnosis or known exposure, and history of herpes. The social history should include asking about country of origin (for TB), recent travel or immigration from the "meningitis belt" of Africa, travel to Midwest or southwest United States (endemic fungal mycoses areas), occupation (school teacher for enterovirus), hobbies (gardener or bird keeper for cryptococcosis), intravenous (IV) drug use (HIV), being incarcerated (TB), sick contacts (enterovirus), sexual activity (HIV, syphilis), and exposure to mosquitoes and ticks. Seasonality also is a factor in the cause of meningitis (eg, enterovirus, mosquito- and tick-borne illnesses are more common in summer). Be sure to review the medication list and ask about antibiotic or NSAID use, and recent immunizations. For treatment purposes, be sure to check for antibiotic allergies.

The classic triad of meningitis symptoms in adults consists of fever, headache, and altered mental status along with physical examination finding of neck stiffness.[20] Ninety-five percent of persons with bacterial meningitis present with 2 of the 4 clinical findings.[21] Other symptoms include photophobia and phonophobia. Other signs include seizures, cranial nerve palsies, and papilledema. Symptoms may develop over several hours or days. Patients with bacterial meningitis are usually quite ill and often present soon after symptom onset. Acute meningitis with duration less than 1 day is almost always a bacterial infection. Patients presenting with symptoms for more than 1 week are very unlikely to have bacterial meningitis (except the bacterial causes that tend to present like aseptic meningitis). In children under the age of 2, symptoms consist of high fever, constant crying, excessive sleepiness, and stiffness in a baby's body and neck.

Certain bacteria, particularly N meningitidis, can cause characteristic skin manifestations, such as petechiae and palpable purpura, In its early phase, it is small, with pinpoint bright red spots covering most of the body; then in its later stage, it becomes raised and purpuric (Fig. 1).

Patients with viral meningitis can also develop a vesicular rash that may cover most of the body or just the arms and the legs. Of the enteroviruses, most meningitis is caused

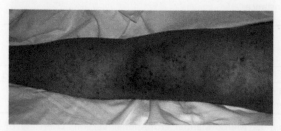

Fig. 1. Rash of meningococcus. (*Courtesy of* Meningitis Research Foundation—www. meningitis.org; Bristol, United Kingdom.)

by the Coxsackie virus, which may also cause small blisters that ulcerate on the hands, feet, and mouth (Figs. 2 and 3). It is not the same as the rash in meningococcal meningitis. Enterovirus meningitis may also present with a sore throat and conjunctivitis. Also, because HSV meningitis is usually concurrent with primary or reactivation of HSV, be sure to check for genital vesicular lesions suggestive of HSV infection.

To assess nuchal rigidity, which seemingly is the most sensitive sign of meningitis compared with Kernig or Brudzinksi signs, passive or active flexion of the neck will usually result in an inability to touch the chin to the chest. The sensitivity of nuchal rigidity is 30%.[22] Brudzinski sign is severe neck stiffness that causes a patient's hips and knees to flex when the neck is flexed. However, Brudzinski sign is neither sensitive nor specific. Difficulty in lateral motion of the neck is also a less reliable finding. Kernig sign is severe stiffness of the hamstrings that causes an inability to straighten the leg when the hip is flexed at 90°. In a prospective study in adults conducted in the United States, having 3 classic meningeal signs did not have good diagnostic value, resulting in sensitivities ranging from 5% to 30%.[23] In another study performed in children, Kernig sign had a similar sensitivity to Brudzinski sign, both around 52%, but Kernig sign had somewhat higher specificity of 95% compared with 77%. The tests did not yield any better results in the subsets of children with moderate or severe meningeal inflammation, nor in relation to any of the causative pathogens.[24]

DIAGNOSTIC EVALUATION

The peripheral WBC count is usually elevated, with a shift toward immature forms; however, severe infection or viral infection can induce leukopenia, thrombocytopenia, and

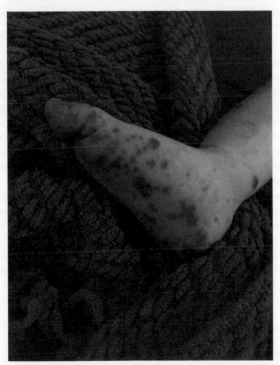

Fig. 2. Rash of Coxsackie virus infection (hand, foot, and mouth disease). (*Courtesy of* S. Dini, MPH, PA-C and her 18-month old son, Atlanta, GA.)

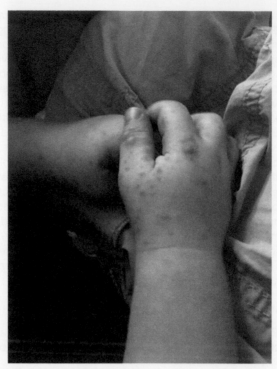

Fig. 3. Rash of Coxsackie virus infection (hand, foot, and mouth disease). (*Courtesy of* S. Dini, MPH, PA-C and her 18-month old son, Atlanta GA.)

hepatitis (especially lymphocytic choriomeningitis virus, Epstein-Barr virus, cytomegalovirus, mumps, and some arboviruses). Blood cultures are often positive and can be useful if CSF cannot be obtained before the administration of antimicrobials. Approximately 50% of patients with bacterial meningitis have positive blood cultures, less likely in patients with meningococcal infection.[20] In one study, blood cultures were positive in 74% of cases and in 57% to 68% of cases with negative CSF cultures.[25] Prior administration of antimicrobials tends to have minimal effects on the chemistry and cytology findings but can reduce the Gram stain and culture.[22,26] However, a pathogen can still be cultured from the CSF in most patients up to several hours after the administration of antimicrobial agents, with the possible exception of meningococcus.[26] This issue was addressed in a review of 128 children with bacterial meningitis in whom lumbar puncture (LP) was first performed after initiation of therapy and serial LPs were obtained. Among patients with meningococcal infection, CSF culture was negative in 33% of samples obtained within 1 hour. In contrast, 4 to 10 hours were required before CSF cultures were sterile in patients with pneumococcal meningitis. Group B streptococcal cultures were positive through the first 8 hours after parenteral antibiotics.[25]

The diagnosis of meningitis rests on the CSF examination (Table 3). Opening pressure is usually elevated with bacterial meningitis. In untreated bacterial meningitis, there is CSF pleocytosis (increased CSF WBC count), usually in the range of 1000 to 5000 cells/mm^3 with neutrophilic predominance.[27] With viral meningitis, the CSF WBC is usually in the several hundreds with a lymphocytic predominance. Protein can be elevated with meningitis, which suggests that there is a blood-brain barrier injury. CSF glucose is usually low (hypoglycorrhachia) as the bacteria metabolize it.

Table 3
Cerebrospinal fluid findings

Test	Bacterial	Viral	Fungal	Tubercular	Noninfectious/malignant
Opening pressure	Elevated	Usually normal	Variable	Variable	Variable
WBC count	>1000 per mm^3	100s–2000 per mm^3	Variable	Variable	Increased
Cell differential	Predominance of PMNs	Predominance of lymphocytes[a]	Predominance of lymphocytes	Predominance of lymphocytes	Variable
Protein	Mild to marked elevation	Normal to elevated	Elevated	Elevated	Elevated
Glucose	Low	Normal	Low	Low	Variable
CSF-to-serum glucose ratio[b]	Normal to marked decrease	Usually normal	Low	Low	Low

a PMNs, polymorphonuclear leukocytes, may predominate early in the course.
b Normal is 0.6.

Other studies include serum glucose, which is compared with the CSF glucose. If the ratio is less than 60%, it is suggestive of bacterial meningitis.[28] Diabetic patients may have elevated CSF glucose, and therefore, the ratio tends to be a more accurate marker than CSF glucose alone. CSF bacterial antigen testing is generally not helpful because it is 30% to 40% sensitive; however, it is around 95% specific. The Gram stain seems to correlate better with bacterial infection.[29,30] Additional CSF testing can include bacterial, viral, acid-fast bacilli (AFB) and fungal cultures; cryptococcal antigen; nucleic acid tests (eg, polymerase chain reaction [PCR]) for enterovirus, HSV-1 and -2, VZV, and M tuberculosis; WNV serology or PCR, and Venereal Disease Research Laboratory test for syphilis. Unfortunately, bacterial culture is not finalized before 3 to 5 days, and viral cultures can take up to 7 to 10 days to be resulted and generally are not helpful to affect therapy in real time. Similarly, because fungal and AFB testing are not finalized for 4 and 6 weeks, respectively, these are not helpful with treatment in real time either.

Serum procalcitonin, C-reactive protein (CRP), and CSF lactate testing can also be helpful. An elevated procalcitonin level of greater than 0.5 ng/mL is 99% sensitive and 83% specific at helping to diagnose bacterial meningitis because it is not elevated in viral meningitis.[20] Patients with bacterial meningitis have an elevated CRP with a median value of 13 ng/mL compared with viral meningitis of 0.03 ng/mL. Elevated CSF lactate greater than 35 mg/dL was shown to have a sensitivity of 93% and a specificity of 96% for bacterial meningitis if obtained before antibiotics.[3]

Management

Treatment of bacterial meningitis begins with empiric antibiotics immediately after LP but before neuroimaging, if ordered, resulting in improved morbidity.[31,32] One study that evaluated appropriate management of meningitis patients according to Infectious Diseases Society of America guidelines showed that the clinicians followed the guidelines poorly, mostly because antibiotic choice is often incorrect, corticosteroids were rarely administered, and there is an overutilization of neuroimaging.[33]

If patients have signs suggesting increased intracranial pressure or a mass effect, immediate LP is deferred and computed tomographic scan of the head is ordered. For example, patients with the following should have LP deferred[27]:

1. Focal neurologic defects (hemiparesis)
2. Papilledema
3. Deteriorating consciousness
4. Seizure within 1 week of presentation
5. Immunocompromised state
6. History of cerebral spinal disease (eg, mass, stroke, infection)

If LP is delayed or deferred, blood cultures should be obtained and antimicrobial therapy should be administered empirically before the imaging study, followed as soon as possible by the LP. However, if the patient does not have risk factors for increased intracranial pressure (see list above), then imaging is not recommended. Prompt initiation of empiric antibacterial therapy as appropriate for patient age and condition should be started (see Table 1). Steroids, usually dexamethasone, should be administered to decrease brain and cranial nerve inflammation and intracranial pressure. Dexamethasone should be initiated 10 to 20 minutes before, or at least at the same time as, the first antimicrobial dose. The recommended dose is 0.15 mg/kg IV every 6 hours × 2 to 4 days. Dexamethasone is not recommended for neonates.[27] In one study conducted in the Netherlands, dexamethasone significantly reduced mortality (7% vs 15% [placebo]), with the most significant effect seen in patients with *S pneumoniae* meningitis.[34] A recent *Cochrane Database Review*, published in 2015, showed that there were lower rates of hearing loss in patients who received dexamethasone.[35] After identification of the pathogen and determination of susceptibilities, antibiotics can be narrowed.

ANTIMICROBIAL RECOMMENDATIONS

Antibiotics must be bactericidal for the suspected bacteria and must be able to penetrate the blood-brain barrier. After 24 hours of appropriate antibiotic treatment initiation, patients are rendered noninfectious. The following antibiotics are recommended (see Table 1).

Other Meningitis Treatment

Cryptococcosis: Antifungal treatment usually deferred to expert infectious diseases (ID) consultation.
Tuberculous: Antitubercular treatment usually deferred to expert ID consultation.
    Herpes or VZV: Acyclovir 10 mg/kg every 8 hours for 10 days total; may change to oral acyclovir or valacyclovir when able to tolerate oral medications.

PREVENTING BACTERIAL MENINGITIS
Antimicrobial Chemoprophylaxis

The primary means for prevention of sporadic meningococcal disease is antimicrobial chemoprophylaxis of close contacts, including health care personnel or infected persons who have had contact with the patient 7 days before symptom onset. Chemoprophylaxis should be administered as soon as possible, ideally less than 24 hours after identification of the index patient.[11] For adults, rifampin 600 mg orally twice a day × 2 days, ciprofloxacin 500 mg orally once, or ceftriaxone 250 mg intramuscularly once are 90% to 95% effective in reducing nasopharyngeal carriage of *N meningitidis* and are all acceptable antimicrobial agents for chemoprophylaxis.

Vaccination

N meningitidis vaccine
Two types of meningitis vaccines (conjugate [Menactra and Menveo] and polysaccharide [Menomune]) protect against 4 serogroups (A, C, W-135, Y) of meningococcal disease. There are 2 additional vaccines that protect against serotype B (Bexsero and Trumenba). Serogroups B, C, and Y are the major causes of meningococcal disease in the United States, each being responsible for approximately one-third of cases.[11] All are about 85% to 90% effective in preventing meningococcal disease.
    The current meningococcal vaccine (A, C, W-135, Y) recommendations are as follows[36]:

1. For infants as young as 6 weeks who are at risk for meningococcal disease because of having complement deficiency, functional or anatomic asplenia, including sickle cell disease, or who have HIV infection
2. All children ages 11 to 18 years old
3. People aged 19 to 21 years old who are first-year college students living in residence halls
4. Traveling or being a resident of countries where meningococcal disease is endemic
5. Being present during an outbreak
6. Microbiologists routinely exposed to isolates of *N meningitidis*

7. As of June 2016, the American Committee on Immunization Practices has recommended that all HIV-infected patients be vaccinated

Certain persons aged 10 years and older who are at increased risk for meningococcal disease should receive the serotype B vaccine. These persons include the following[37]:

1. Persons with persistent complement component deficiencies
2. Persons with anatomic or functional asplenia
3. Microbiologists routinely exposed to isolates of *N meningitidis*
4. Persons identified as at increased risk because of a serogroup B meningococcal disease outbreak

S pneumoniae and H influenzae Vaccines

As stated previously, with the increased acceptance and use of pneumococcal and *H influenzae* vaccines, meningitis due to these causes has decreased significantly.

Posttest

How did you do?

1. What is the most common etiologic agent causing meningitis in the United States?
   Viral infections are diagnosed more commonly than bacterial infections, by a magnitude of 10, and enterovirus is the most commonly reported viral cause.
2. What is the most common bacterium that causes meningitis in the United States?
   Streptococcus pneumoniae
3. What antibiotics should be initiated for suspected bacterial meningitis in the United States for adult patients with no past medical history?
   Vancomycin and Ceftriaxone or Cefotaxime

SUMMARY

Meningitis remains a serious personal and public health problem both worldwide and in the United States. It can range from self-limiting and benign with viral meningitis to life-threatening with serious sequelae as in bacterial meningitis. It is important for clinicians to remain vigilant and look for signs and symptoms of meningitis. One last important recommendation is that if meningitis is even remotely in the differential diagnosis, it is important to order the LP and the appropriate antibiotics because treatment can be de-escalated if the CSF looks nonbacterial. With prompt recognition and initiation of antibiotics, patients can recover more quickly with less adverse events.

REFERENCES

1. Brooks R, Woods CW, Benjamin DK Jr, et al. Increased case fatality rate associated with outbreaks of Neisseria meningitidis infection, compared with sporadic meningococcal disease in the US, 1994-2002. Clin Infect Dis 2006;43(1):49–54.
2. Medscape Viral Meningitis: Wan C, Singh NN. Available at: http://emedicine. medscape.com/article/1168529-overview. Accessed Sepetember 21, 2016.
3. Bahr NC, Boulware DR. Methods of rapid diagnosis for the etiology of meningitis in adults. Biomark Med 2014;8(9):1085–103.
4. Kupila L, Vuorinen T, Vainionpaa R, et al. Etiology of aseptic meningitis and encephalitis in an adult population. Neurology 2006;66(1):75–80.
5. Thigpen MC, Whitney CG, Messonnier NE, et al. Bacterial meningitis in the United States, 1998–2007. N Engl J Med 2011;364:2016–25.

6. Brouwer MC, Tunkel AR, van de Beek D. Epidemiology, diagnosis, and antimicrobial treatment of acute bacterial meningitis. Clin Microbiol Rev 2010;23(3): 467–92.

7. Whitney CG, Farley MM, Hadler J, et al. Decline in invasive pneumococcal disease after the introduction of protein-polysaccharide conjugate vaccine. N Engl J Med 2003;348(18):1737–46.

8. Lepoutre A, Varon E, Georges S, et al. Impact of the pneumococcal conjugate vaccines on invasive pneumococcal disease in France, 2001-2012. Vaccine 2015;33(2):359–66.

9. Sangil A, Xercavins M, Rodriguez-Carballeira M, et al. Impact of vaccination on invasive pneumococcal disease in adults with focus on the immunosuppressed. J Infect 2015;71(4):422–7.

10. Cartwright KA, Stuart JM, Jones DM, et al. The Stonehouse survey: nasopharyngeal carriage of meningococci and Neisseria lactamica. Epidemiol Infect 1987; 99(3):591–601.

11. Centers for Disease Control and Prevention. Epidemiology and prevention of vaccine-preventable diseases. In: Hamborsky J, Kroger A, Wolfe S, editors. Meningococcal Disease. 13th edition. Washington, DC: Public Health Foundation; 2015.

12. García-Pando CP, Stanton MC, Diggle PJ, et al. Soil dust aerosols and wind as predictors of seasonal meningitis incidence in Niger. Environ Health Perspect 2014;122(7):679–86.

13. Centers for Disease Control and Prevention, Viral meningitis. Available at: http://www.cdc.gov/meningitis/viral.html. Accessed September 23, 2016.

14. Shelburne C, Statler M. Meningitis: distinguishing the benign from the serious. JAAPA 2008;21(4):54–9.

15. Becerra JCM, Sieber R, Martinetti G, et al. Infection of the central nervous system caused by varicella zoster virus reactivation: a retrospective case series study. Int J Infect Dis 2013;17(7):e529–34.

16. Rafaillidis PI, Kapaskelis A, Falagas ME. Cytomegalovirus meningitis in an immunocompetent patient. Med Sci Monit 2007;13(9):CS107–9.

17. Marx GE, Chan ED. Tuberculous meningitis: diagnosis and treatment overview. Tuberc Res Treat 2011;2011:1–9.

18. Bihanic T, Harrison TS. Cryptococcal meningitis. Br Med Bull 2004;72(1):99–118.

19. Rodríguez SC, Olquin AM, Miralles CP, et al. Characteristics of meningitis caused by Ibuprofen: report of 2 cases with recurrent episodes and review of the literature. Medicine 2006;85(4):214–20.

20. Meningitis. Hasbun R. Medscape Web site. Available at: http://emedicine.medscape.com/article/232915-overview. Accessed May 31, 2016.

21. van de Beek D, de Gans J, Spanjaard L, et al. Clinical features and prognostic factors in adults with bacterial meningitis. N Engl J Med 2004;351(18):1849–59.

22. Tunkel A, editor. Up To Date. Waltham (MA): Up to Date. Literature review current through; 2016. Meningitis.

23. Thomas KE, Hasbun R, Jekel J, et al. The diagnostic accuracy of Kernig's sign, Brudzinski's sign, and nuchal rigidity in adults with suspected meningitis. Clin Infect Dis 2002;35(1):46.

24. Bilavsky E, Leibovitz E, Elkon-Tamir E, et al. The diagnostic accuracy of the 'classic meningeal signs' in children with suspected bacterial meningitis. Eur J Emerg Med 2013;20(5):361–3.

25. Kanegaye JT, Soliemanzadeh P, Bradley JS. Lumbar puncture in pediatric bacterial meningitis: defining the time interval for recovery of cerebrospinal fluid pathogens after parenteral antibiotic pretreatment. Pediatrics 2001;108:1169–74.

26. Geiseler PJ, Nelson KE, Levin S, et al. Community-acquired purulent meningitis: a review of 1,316 cases during the antibiotic era, 1954-1976. Rev Infect Dis 1980; 2(5):725–45.

27. Tunkel AR, Hartman BJ, Kaplan SL, et al. Practice guidelines for the management of bacterial meningitis. Clin Infect Dis 2004;39:1267–84.

28. Greenlee JE. Merck Manual Professional Version. Overview of meningitis. Available at: http://www.merckmanuals.com/professional/neurologic-disorders/meningitis/overview-of-meningitis. Accessed September 23, 2016.

29. Perkins MD, Mirrett S, Reller LB. Rapid bacterial antigen testing is not clinically useful. J Clin Microbiol 1995;33(6):1486–91.

30. Mein J, Lum G. CSF bacterial antigen detection tests offer no advantage over Gram's stain in the diagnosis of bacterial meningitis. Pathology 1999;31(1):67–9.

31. Feldman WE, Ginsburg CM, McCracken GH Jr. Relation of concentrations of Haemophilus influenza type B in cerebrospinal fluid to late sequelae of patients with meningitis. J Pediatr 1982;100(2):209–12.

32. Lebel MH, McCracken GH Jr. Delayed cerebrospinal fluid sterilization and adverse outcome of bacterial meningitis in infants and children. Pediatrics 1989;83(2):161–7.

33. Chia D, Yavari Y, Kirsanov E, et al. Adherence to standard of care in the diagnosis and treatment of suspected bacterial meningitis. Am J Med Qual 2015;30(6): 539–42.

34. De Gans J, van de Beek D. Dexamethasone in adults with bacterial meningitis. N Engl J Med 2002;347(20):1549–56.

35. Brouwer MC, McIntyre P, Prasad K, et al. Corticosteroids for acute bacterial meningitis. Cochrane Database Syst Rev 2015;(9):CD004405.

36. CDC Prevention and Control of Meningococcal Disease Recommendations of the Advisory Committee on Immunization Practices (ACIP). MMWR Recomm Rep 2013;62(No. RR-#):1–28. Available at: http://www.cdc.gov/mmwr/pdf/rr/rr6202.pdf.

37. CDC, Folaranmi T, Rubin L, et al. Use of serogroup B meningococcal vaccines in persons aged ≥10 years at increased risk for serogroup B meningococcal disease: recommendations of the Advisory Committee on Immunization Practices, 2015. MMWR Recomm Rep 2015;62(22):608.

Current Diagnosis and Management of Urinary Tract Infections

Tia Solh, PA-C, MT(ASCP), MPAS[a],*,
Rebekah Thomas, PA-C, PharmD, BCPS, BC-ADM[b],
Christopher Roman, PA-C, MA, MMS[c]

KEYWORDS

- Urinary tract infection • UTI • Cystitis • Pyelonephritis • Complicated UTI
- Asymptomatic bacteriuria

KEY POINTS

- Urinary tract infections (UTIs) are classified as complicated and uncomplicated, which dictates their management; a majority of UTIs are uncomplicated and occur in previously healthy, nonpregnant women.
- Urinalysis results must be interpreted carefully, because several indicators, if used individually, do not have adequate sensitivity or specificity for confirmation of UTI.
- First-line agents for the empirical treatment of acute, uncomplicated cystitis in the United States are nitrofurantoin, trimethoprim/sulfamethoxazole, and fosfomycin.
- Asymptomatic bacteriuria does not require treatment in most patients, with the exceptions of pregnancy and prior to urologic procedures.
- Asymptomatic candiduria is not an immediate indication for treatment in most patients but should be investigated further.

INTRODUCTION

The term, *urinary tract infection*, encompasses a broad spectrum of infections along the urinary tract, from simple cystitis to severe pyelonephritis. UTIs are the most commonly encountered bacterial infection in the ambulatory setting in the United States.[1] Although most UTIs are uncomplicated, they are also a leading cause of gram-negative sepsis. The estimated annual cost of treatment of UTIs exceeds $2

Disclosure Statement: The authors have no financial conflict of interest related to this article.
[a] Department of Physician Assistant Studies, Mercer University, 3001 Mercer University Drive, Atlanta, GA 30341, USA; [b] Department of Physician Assistant Studies, Philadelphia College of Osteopathic Medicine, 625 Old Peachtree Road Northwest, Suwanee, GA 30024, USA; [c] Physician Assistant Program, Butler University, 4600 Sunset Avenue, Indianapolis, IN 46208, USA
* Corresponding author.
E-mail address: Solh_tm@mercer.edu

Physician Assist Clin 2 (2017) 191–205
http://dx.doi.org/10.1016/j.cpha.2016.12.003
2405-7991/17/© 2016 Elsevier Inc. All rights reserved.
physicianassistant.theclinics.com

billion in the United States.[1] This article reviews the epidemiology, risk factors, pathophysiology, and current diagnosis and treatment of UTIs.

DEFINITIONS
Urinary Tract Infection

A UTI results from microbial invasion of the urinary tract, which is normally sterile.[1] Lower tract infections result from invasion of the urethra and bladder, respectively termed urethritis and cystitis. Upper tract infections involve the ureters and kidney, respectively termed ureteritis and pyelonephritis. Both lower tract infections and upper tract infections can be considered uncomplicated or complicated.

Uncomplicated Urinary Tract Infection

A majority of UTIs are uncomplicated and are defined as infection in otherwise healthy, nonpregnant women with urinary tracts of normal structure and function.[2] By age 24, 1 in 3 women are treated for a UTI.[1] Uncomplicated UTIs can rarely occur in men, but a vast majority of urinary tract infections in men are considered complicated.[3]

Complicated Urinary Tract Infection

UTIs are considered complicated when they are associated with any underlying condition that increases the risk of treatment failure. Conditions associated with complicated UTIs include[2]

- Pregnancy
- Diabetes
- HIV
- Immunosuppression
- Infection with multidrug-resistant pathogen
- Functional or anatomic abnormalities of the urinary tract
- Renal insufficiency
- Renal transplant
- Obstruction of the urinary tract (eg, calculi or stenosis)
- Presence of instrumentation (eg, indwelling urinary catheter, stent, or nephrostomy tube)

Recurrent Urinary Tract Infection

Recurrent UTIs are defined as 2 uncomplicated infections within 6 months or as 3 infections within 12 months, with clearance of the initial infection demonstrated by negative urine culture. Despite adequate antimicrobial treatment of the initial infection, a patient has a 25% probability of developing a second UTI within 6 months and 46% probability of recurrence over 12 months.[1]

Asymptomatic Bacteriuria

Asymptomatic bacteriuria is defined as the presence of bacteria in an appropriately collected urine sample from a patient without any urinary symptoms or signs of a UTI.[3] It usually does not warrant antimicrobial treatment except in special populations, as discussed later.

Pyuria

Pyuria is defined as the presence of an increased amount of polymorphonuclear lymphocytes in the urine and indicates inflammation of the urinary tract.[3] It is not necessarily an indication of a UTI, as discussed later.

PATHOGENS

Escherichia coli causes 75% to 95% of uncomplicated cystitis and pyelonephritis across all settings and all age groups.[4,5] *E coli* is estimated to be responsible for 65% of hospital-acquired infections and 47% of health care–associated infections in the United States.[5] Some of these strains have an enhanced ability to cause UTIs due to several virulent factors, including a type of pili that promotes biofilm formation, and are thus termed uropathogenic *E coli* (UPEC).[1] Multidrug resistance of UPEC has increased and is becoming increasingly common in community-acquired UTIs.[1,5]

Other members of the Enterobacteriaceae family, such as *Klebsiella pneumoniae* and *Proteus mirabilis*, as well as gram-positive organisms, such as *Staphylococcus saprophyticus* and *Enterococcus faecalis*, are less frequent causes of UTIs.[6] Risk factors associated with infection with these pathogens include urinary catheters, obstruction, male gender, and recurrent UTI.[5]

PATHOPHYSIOLOGY AND RISK FACTORS

Several risk factors account for the vast majority of UTIs. These include

- Female gender
- Behavioral factors
- Microbial and immune system properties
- Anatomic abnormalities
- Iatrogenic causes

Because an understanding of these risk factors follows directly from the pathophysiology of these infections, this section considers each risk factor separately with an explanation of the relevant pathogenesis for that topic.

A vast majority of UTIs are ascending infections that begin with the colonization of the urethra with fecal microbes. These subsequently ascend up the urethra and into the bladder. Further progression of this infection can manifest with bacteremia and/ or ascent of the pathogens up the ureters and into the kidneys (pyelonephritis). Additional modes of acquisition for UTI can include hematogenous or, rarely, lymphatic introduction of microbes into the urinary tract, although both of these are much less common than the ascending route.[7] Importantly, hematogenous spread infrequently occurs with the gram-negative microbes that typically cause UTI. Instead, organisms, such as *Candida*, enterococci, *Salmonella* spp, and *Staphylococcus aureus*, are the common pathogens for UTI after bloodstream infection.[7] Because they are uncommon uropathogens, isolation of 1 of these organisms from the urine of a hospitalized or critically ill patient warrants an investigation for a bacteremic source that has seeded the kidneys. Because these pathogens are also frequent etiologic agents of infective endocarditis, blood cultures as well as an echocardiogram, preferably transesophageal, should be performed.

Female Gender

A majority of UTIs occur in female patients, and up to 50% of women require treatment of a UTI by age 32.[8] This risk is mediated through several factors, including

- Short (approximately 4-cm) urethras compared with male patients (approximately 20 cm), allowing for quicker ascent of pathogens to the bladder
- Heavy colonization of the anogenital area with potentially pathogenic (eg, *E coli*) as well as commensal (eg, lactobacilli) bacteria

- In postmenopausal women, the lack of estrogen can decrease native flora and decrease local immune function[9,10]

Behavioral Factors

Sexual intercourse is frequently associated with UTI, with the following factors identified in research studies:

- Frequency of intercourse[11]
- Use of spermidicides, which modifies the genitourinary flora[12,13]
- New sexual partner within the past year[13]
- Men having sex with men; they seem to have more frequent UTIs, presumably due to anogenital flora introduced during anal intercourse[14]

Although not definitively proved, several recent case-control studies performed outside the United States indicate that certain cultural practices, such as wiping from back to front after defecating and washing the perineum from back to front, may increase the likelihood of developing UTI.[15–18] Precoital and postcoital voiding may decrease the urethral bacterial levels and reduce the risk of UTI.[19] There is a paucity of data, however, on all of these items.[6]

Microbial and Immunologic Factors

Many of the common pathogens in UTI have characteristics that allow for survival and proliferation within the urogenital tract.[20] As discussed previously, alterations in urogenital flora increase the risk of UTI. These may occur with administration of antimicrobial agents that alter or eliminate the normal flora[21] while also increasing bacterial drug resistance within the host for several months.[22] The immunologic effects of low estrogen are discussed previously, but other immunocompromised states also experience increased risk of UTI due to host inability to control colonization and invasion of pathogens.[23,24] Both a history of previous UTI and maternal history of UTI for female patients are risk factors for subsequent UTI; whether this is genetic or otherwise heritable has not been determined.[13] Recurrent UTIs are thought to be due to bacterial invasion of the bladder mucosa, followed by the formation of intracellular reservoirs that are shielded from antibiotics and host defenses.[1]

Anatomic Abnormalities

The presence of several anatomic abnormalities can contribute to UTI:

- Prostatic enlargement or inflammation
- Renal calculi, which can obstruct the renal outflow tract or can themselves become infected
- Urinary tract obstruction and/or retention, which increases bacterial levels in the urine
- Vesicoureteral reflux, which facilitates the ascent of pathogens to the upper urinary tract

Iatrogenic Causes

Up to 97% of nosocomial UTIs are directly attributed to urinary catheterization.[25] The duration of catheter placement is the greatest predictor of UTI, with the risk of bacteriuria increasing by approximately 5% per day.[26,27] Once introduced to the surface of the catheter, bacteria colonize the instrument and form a biofilm. The pathogens then move proximally and eventually enter the bladder. Extraluminal contamination accounts for approximately 66% of catheter-associated UTIs, whereas intraluminal infections arise in the other 34%.[28] As a result, the microorganisms identified in these infections are much more varied than those found in non–catheter-associated UTIs.[28] UTIs may arise after other instrumentation of the urinary tract (eg, cystoscopy),[29] but these procedures are performed less commonly than catheterization.

DIAGNOSTIC EVALUATION
History and Physical Examination

Diagnosis of UTI begins with a thorough medical history, assessing for

- Risk factors of UTI
- Fever
- Urinary urgency and frequency
- Dysuria
- Abdominal pain
- Vaginal discharge and irritation
- Changes in urine odor, color, or consistency

Physical examination should include assessment for suprapubic tenderness, flank pain, and costovertebral angle (CVA) tenderness, which aid in the differentiation between a lower tract infection and an upper tract infection. Patients with cystitis usually present with suprapubic tenderness and complaints of lower abdominal pain and/or pressure, whereas patients with pyelonephritis commonly present with the following signs and symptoms:

- Nausea
- Vomiting
- Fever (temperature >100.4°F)
- Chills
- Low back pain
- Flank pain
- CVA tenderness

Patients complaining of vaginal discharge should receive a pelvic examination to rule out cervicitis, pelvic inflammatory disease, or vaginitis as a source of dysuria. The presence of dysuria and urinary frequency without vaginal symptoms increases the probability of UTI to 90%, whereas the added presence of vaginal symptoms decreases the probability to 30%.[30]

Urinalysis

Accurate diagnosis requires an appropriately collected urine specimen that minimizes contamination. Midstream clean-catch, straight catheter collection, and suprapubic aspiration are accepted techniques. Urinalysis is commonly performed by dipstick, and the following are common indicators[1,2]:

- Hematuria
- Nitrite
- Leukocyte esterase
- Low-grade proteinuria

The presence of red blood cells, nitrite, and leukocyte esterase in a patient with suggestive symptoms is strongly predictive of a UTI.[1] If microscopy is performed, the finding of 10 or more leukocytes per high-power field strongly correlates with UTIs.[2] White blood cell casts on microscopy confirm an upper tract infection.

The finding of yeast occurs in less than 1% of urine specimens, and its significance ranges from contamination to an indication of life-threatening, invasive candidiasis. Therefore, this finding should not be treated empirically and should always be investigated further by collecting a second urine sample.[31]

Leukocyte Esterase

Leukocyte esterase assesses for pyuria. Pyuria reflects inflammation in the genitourinary tract but it does not determine infectious etiology. It is present in many conditions, including asymptomatic bacteriuria, urinary infection, and interstitial nephritis, in the presence of an indwelling urinary device and after a urologic surgical procedure.[3] Therefore, a positive finding of leukocyte esterase alone is not diagnostic of UTI and is not an indication for antimicrobial treatment in and of itself.[32]

Nitrite

The Enterobacteriaceae family, consisting of gram-negative bacilli, converts urinary nitrates to nitrites, and a positive nitrite result is reflective of their presence. The dipstick nitrite test has a reported specificity of up to 98%. Not all urinary pathogens reduce nitrates to nitrites, however, and a meta-analysis of 70 studies found that the overall sensitivity of the urine dipstick for nitrites in predicting urinary infection was 45% to 60%.[33] Therefore, a negative nitrite result does not rule out infection and should be interpreted with caution in a patient with urinary symptoms.

Urine Culture

A positive urinalysis in a patient with signs and symptoms of an uncomplicated UTI is usually sufficient for diagnosis, but a urine culture with susceptibility testing should be performed during pregnancy, empirical treatment failure, and when an upper tract infection, complicated UTI, or recurrent UTI is suspected. The diagnostic criteria for asymptomatic bacteriuria, uncomplicated cystitis, and catheter-associated UTI are detailed in Table 1.

Table 1
Diagnostic criteria for asymptomatic bacteriuria, uncomplicated cystitis, and catheter-associated urinary tract infection based on urine culture

Asymptomatic Bacteriuria[3]	Uncomplicated Cystitis[1]	Catheter-Associated Urinary Tract Infection[32]
2 Consecutive voided urine specimens in women with $\geq 10^5$ CFU/mL of the same bacterial strain	$\geq 10^3$ CFU/mL in a urine specimen in a patient with signs or symptoms of a UTI	$\geq 10^3$ CFU/mL in a urine specimen in a patient with signs or symptoms of a UTI
1 Voided urine specimen in men with $\geq 10^5$ CFU/mL of 1 bacterial species		
1 Catheterized urine specimen in women or men with $\geq 10^2$ CFU/mL of 1 bacterial species		

Abbreviation: CFU, colony-forming unit.
Data from Refs.[1,3,32]

Blood Cultures

Blood cultures should be reserved for patients with suspected sepsis secondary to UTI as well as for hospitalized patients suspected of UTI due to hematogenous spread. Obtaining blood cultures on admission for patients with complicated UTI requiring hospitalization may be of value, because a recent study of 800 hospitalized patients showed that in a small percentage of patients, the uropathogens responsible for bacteremia were isolated from the blood but not the urine.[34] In addition, lack of response to antimicrobial therapy during hospitalization should prompt repeat blood cultures, and possibly imaging studies, to rule out a stone, mass, or other obstruction as a persistent nidus of infection (eg, an infected obstructing renal calculus or an intra-renal abscess).[30]

Imaging

Imaging is usually unnecessary for episodes of cystitis and pyelonephritis, except in cases of anatomic abnormalities or suspected obstruction. Indications for the use of imaging in the setting of pyelonephritis include[2]

- Unresponsiveness to antibiotic therapy after 48 hours to 72 hours of treatment
- Diabetes
- Nephrolithiasis
- History of urologic surgery

CT is the imaging study of choice for the detection of calculi, abscesses, hemorrhage, and obstruction; however, renal and pelvic ultrasound is preferred for patients in whom contrast or ionizing radiation is hazardous and can also identify abnormalities, such as calculi, hydronephrosis, hydroureter, proximal obstruction of the ureter, and congenital anomalies, such as ureterocele, although ultrasound is less sensitive than CT.[35] MRI should not be considered an initial imaging source due to decreased consistency identifying stones.[2,3]

TREATMENT
Optimal Empirical Antimicrobial Treatment

Several factors necessitate consideration when selecting an appropriate empirical antimicrobial agent. These factors include common causative pathogens, local resistance patterns, severity of illness, and collateral damage. Collateral damage refers to adverse events associated with the use of antimicrobial therapy, such as the potential for colonization with multidrug-resistant organisms when using broad-spectrum agents.[4,6]

When choosing an antimicrobial agent based on local resistance patterns, resistance percentages of causative microorganisms should be less than 20% to consider an agent adequate for empirical treatment of a lower UTI and less than 10% for treatment of an upper UTI.[4] Patterns of resistance vary with patient population and geographic regions within the United States, and it is prudent for practitioners to be familiar with their respective community-based or institution-based antibiogram. Due to high prevalence of resistance with amoxicillin, it is inappropriate for empirical treatment of cystitis.[4] Empirical first-line and alternative agents for the treatment of uncomplicated cystitis are listed in Table 2. Oral β-lactams, nitrofurantoin, trimethoprim, and trimethoprim/sulfamethoxazole have been deemed inadequate empirical therapy for complicated UTI and pyelonephritis due to high resistance patterns.[1,2,4]

After obtaining a urine culture with susceptibility testing, women requiring hospitalization for complicated UTI or pyelonephritis should initially be treated with IV

Table 2
Empirical antimicrobial agents for the treatment of acute uncomplicated cystitis

Drug	Efficacy	Dosing	Side Effects	Considerations	Resistance	Dosing Adjustment for Renal Impairment
Nitrofurantoin monohydrate/ macrocrystals	First-line agent	100 mg by mouth twice a day × 5 d	Nausea, vomiting, diarrhea, hypersensitivity reaction	Rare cases of pulmonary fibrosis in long-term use	Low resistance rates	Use not recommended when CrCl <60 mL/min
Trimethoprim/ sulfamethoxazole	First-line agent	1 double strength tablet by mouth twice a day × 3 d	Nausea, vomiting; Stevens-Johnson syndrome in rare cases	Increased bleeding risk with warfarin Risk of hyperkalemia with low GFR or when administered with ACE inhibitor, ARB, or aldosterone antagonist	Avoid when local resistance patterns exceed 20%	CrCl 15–30 mL/min: Administer 50% of recommended dose. Do not use if CrCl <15 mL/min.
Fosfomycin	First-line agent; less efficacious than other first-line agents	3 g by mouth × 1	Nausea, diarrhea, vaginitis	Symptom improvement within days of treatment	Low resistance rates	No adjustment required
Ciprofloxacin	Second-line agent; per FDA, benefits of fluoroquinolone use for uncomplicated cystitis do not outweigh the risks	250 mg by mouth twice a day × 3 d	Nausea, vomiting, diarrhea, headache	Risk of C difficile colitis, tendonitis, tendon rupture, myopathy, neuropathy, depression, hallucinations, suicidal ideation	Increasing resistance across the United States	Adjustment needed when CrCl <30 mL/min

Abbreviations: ACE, angiotensin-converting enzyme; ARB, angiotensin receptor blocker; CrCl, creatinine clearance; GFR, glomerular filtration rate.
Data from Gupta K, Hooton TM, Naber KG, et al. International clinical practice guidelines for the treatment of acute uncomplicated cystitis and pyelonephritis in women: a 2010 update by the Infectious Diseases Society of America and the European Society for Microbiology and Infectious Diseases. Clin Infect Dis 2011;52(5):e103–20; and Hooton TM. Clinical practice. Uncomplicated urinary tract infection. N Engl J Med 2012;366(11):1028–37.

antimicrobials. Potential empirical regimens, which should be chosen based on local resistance patterns, include monotherapy with a fluoroquinolone (eg, levofloxacin), aminoglycoside (eg, gentamicin), third-generation cephalosporin (eg, ceftriaxone or ceftazidime), or carbapenem (eg, ertapenem) or combination therapy with an amino-glycoside and third-generation cephalosporin (eg, gentamicin plus ceftazidime).[4] The initial antimicrobial regimen should then be tailored once susceptibility results are known.

Cases of uncomplicated cystitis caused by extended-spectrum β-lactamase (ESBL) producing Enterobacteriaceae may be treated the same as cases caused by non-ESBL organisms, if susceptibilities and local resistance patterns are known. Complicated UTIs caused by ESBL-producing organisms require a carbapenem, such as meropenem.[36]

Asymptomatic Bacteriuria

Antibiotic therapy for asymptomatic bacteriuria is not indicated, except in pregnancy or if undergoing a urologic procedure. Treatment of asymptomatic bacteriuria is not indicated in the following populations[3]:

- Diabetic women
- Older community-dwelling persons
- Older residents in long-term care facilities
- Patients with spinal cord injury
- Patients with an indwelling urethral catheter

Screening for asymptomatic bacteriuria should be performed prior to invasive uro-logic procedures associated with mucosal bleeding, such as transurethral resection of the prostate (TURP), given the high incidence of bacteremia and sepsis after TURP. Therapy should be initiated the night prior to or immediately before the procedure and can be discontinued immediately after the procedure, or at the time the indwelling urinary catheter is removed postoperatively.[3] The American Urological Association recommends trimethoprim/sulfamethoxazole or a fluoroquinolone as the agent of choice for most procedures introducing instrumentation to the upper tract.[37] Fluoro-quinolones should be used judiciously, however, because in July 2016, the Food and Drug Administration (FDA) issued a revision to its boxed warning for the systemic use of fluoroquinolones after receiving reports of serious side effects affecting 2 or more body systems in the same patient. The FDA warns that the potentially disabling and possibly permanent side effects of fluoroquinolones, which include arthralgias, tendonitis, tendon rupture, myalgias, myopathy, neuropathy, depression, hallucina-tions, and suicidal thoughts, outweigh its benefits for treatment of uncomplicated UTIs.[38] The updated FDA warning does not specifically comment on their use for uro-logic prophylaxis.

Acute Cystitis

First-line agents for the treatment of acute uncomplicated cystitis include nitrofuran-toin, 100 mg twice daily for 5 days, or 1 double-strength tablet of trimethoprim/sulfa-methoxazole, twice daily for 3 days.[4] Trimethoprim/sulfamethoxazole may be used in regions where local resistance levels are lower than 20%; if levels exceed 20%, the use of nitrofurantoin or fosfomycin is recommended.[4] Fosfomycin is given as a single 3-g dose, although it is slightly less efficacious than the other first-line agents.[4,39] Flu-oroquinolones, specifically ciprofloxacin and levofloxacin, should be reserved for pa-tients who cannot tolerate the recommended first-line agents, due to the increased incidence of resistance in *E coli* and the potential for permanently disabling adverse side effects, as discussed later.[4] β-Lactam antibiotics, such as amoxicillin-clavulanate or cefpodoxime, should only be used as second-line agents, in 3-day to 7-day treatment regimens, due to their decreased efficacy and increased frequency of side effects.[4,6,39]

Recurrent Cystitis

The persistence or recurrence of urinary symptoms within 1 week to 2 weeks of treatment of uncomplicated cystitis suggests possible resistance and the need for a broader-spectrum antimicrobial, such as a fluoroquinolone. If the recurrence is more than 1 month after completion of therapy for cystitis, then an alternative first-line agent should be chosen for current management.[6]

Patients who experience recurrent cystitis should undergo a targeted history and physical examination. The history should focus on identifying predisposing or associated factors and determining any modifiable actions that could be undertaken. Physical examination should include evaluation for vaginal pathology and bladder ultrasound or catheterization to assess for residual urinary volume.[40] A urinalysis should be performed to determine the presence of resistant organisms. Patients experiencing persistent, complicated, febrile infection should receive cystoscopic evaluation to assess for structural abnormalities, such as urethral stricture.[40] Cystoscopy is usually unnecessary in women less than 40 years of age and those without risk factors for structural abnormalities and normal imaging studies. Prophylactic antibiotic regimens with trimethoprim/sulfamethoxazole, nitrofurantoin, or cephalexin can provide some benefit but use should be minimized and reflect a patient-initiated approach to therapy.[2] If recurrence continues to persist, then a referral to urology is merited.

Acute Pyelonephritis

Urine culture and susceptibility testing should be obtained in suspected pyelonephritis prior to initiating therapy to aid in the selection of an antibiotic. Patients who do not require hospitalization can be treated with oral ciprofloxacin, 500 mg twice daily for 7 days. An initial 1-time dose of an intravenous (IV) antibiotic, preferably ciprofloxacin or ceftriaxone, can be considered. In susceptible patients, trimethoprim/sulfamethoxazole (1 double-strength tablet), twice daily for 14 days, is an acceptable therapeutic option.[4] Oral β-lactams are not preferred agents for pyelonephritis, because they require 10 days to 14 days of therapy and are less efficacious. Nitrofurantoin is also not a preferred therapy because it undergoes rapid renal excretion resulting in subtherapeutic blood levels and decreased efficacy.[4,40] The empirical outpatient treatment options for acute uncomplicated pyelonephritis are summarized in Table 3.

Indications for inpatient management of pyelonephritis include complicated infection, hemodynamic instability, high fever, pain intolerance, inability to tolerate oral medications and hydration, pregnancy, and comorbidities, because these patients require hospitalization for initial treatment with IV antibiotics. Appropriate parenteral regimens include monotherapy with a fluoroquinolone (eg, levofloxacin), aminoglycoside (eg, gentamicin), third-generation cephalosporin (eg, ceftriaxone or ceftazidime), or carbapenem (eg, meropenem) or combination therapy with an aminoglycoside and third-generation cephalosporin (eg, gentamicin plus ceftriaxone).[2,4]

SPECIAL CLINICAL SITUATIONS
Pregnancy

Early in pregnancy, women should be screened by urine culture for bacteriuria, and positive culture results are an indication for treatment. Asymptomatic bacteriuria

Table 3
Empirical antimicrobial agents for the outpatient treatment of acute uncomplicated pyelonephritis in nonpregnant patients

Drug	Efficacy	Dosing	Resistance
Ciprofloxacin	First-line agent	500 mg by mouth twice a day × 7 d; may be given with or without a 1-time initial 400-mg dose of parenteral ciprofloxacin	If local resistance patterns exceed 10%, supplement regimen with an initial 1-time dose of a long-acting antimicrobial, such as ceftriaxone, 1 g IV × 1.
Levofloxacin	First-line agent	750 mg by mouth once daily × 5 d	If local resistance patterns exceed 10%, supplement regimen with an initial 1-time dose of a long-acting antimicrobial, such as ceftriaxone, 1 g IV × 1.
Trimethoprim/ sulfamethoxazole	Second-line agent due to high rates of resistance	1 Double-strength tablet by mouth twice a day × 14 d	Do not use if local resistance patterns exceed 20%; if resistance is unknown, may supplement regimen with an initial 1-time dose of a long-acting antimicrobial, such as ceftriaxone, 1 g IV × 1.

Data from Gupta K, Hooton TM, Naber KG, et al. International clinical practice guidelines for the treatment of acute uncomplicated cystitis and pyelonephritis in women: a 2010 update by the Infectious Diseases Society of America and the European Society for Microbiology and Infectious Diseases. Clin Infect Dis 2011;52(5):e103–20; and Hooton TM. Clinical practice. Uncomplicated urinary tract infection. N Engl J Med 2012;366(11):1028–37.

and cystitis in pregnancy can be successfully treated as outpatients.[3] Treatment of asymptomatic bacteriuria has been associated with many positive outcomes, including a significant decrease in the subsequent development of pyelonephritis, decreased frequency of low-birth-weight infants and decreased incidence of preterm delivery. Favorable resistance percentages and lack of teratogenic effects makes β-lactams a good option for treatment of UTI during pregnancy.[41] Although it has not been proved in human studies, fluoroquinolones are not recommended during any stage of pregnancy because they have shown toxicity to developing cartilage in animal studies. Nitrofurantoin is not recommended during the first trimester due to its association with many potential adverse outcomes, including neonatal polyneuropathy and fetal anemia.[42] Similarly, practitioners should avoid use of trimethoprim/sulfamethoxazole during the first trimester, because it is associated with neural tube defects, cardiovascular and urinary system defects, and cleft palate.[41] Trimethoprim/sulfamethoxazole and nitrofurantoin are well tolerated during the second and third trimesters but may result in fetal hyperbilirubinemia and neonatal jaundice and kernicterus if used near term.[42] On completing treatment, screening for recurrent bacteriuria is suggested.

Hospitalization, blood and urine cultures, and IV therapy with a third-generation cephalosporin, such as ceftriaxone or cefotaxime, are recommended for the treatment of pyelonephritis during pregnancy.[41,42] Aztreonam, which is also FDA pregnancy category B and administered parenterally, is an acceptable alternative for patients with β-lactam allergies. Gentamicin and other aminoglycosides, due to the potential risk of fetal neurotoxicity and nephrotoxicity, should be reserved for cases where no acceptable alternative agent exists and when the benefits for the mother outweigh the risk to the fetus (eg, in life-threatening cases). When symptom improvement is noted and the patient has been afebrile for 24 hours to 48 hours, it is reasonable to consider transitioning from IV to oral therapy. Treatment should be continued for a total duration of 10 days and a follow-up urine culture should be obtained. After treatment of pyelonephritis, patients should receive prophylaxis with cephalexin daily throughout the remainder of the pregnancy and for 4 weeks to 6 weeks postpartum. Patients who fail to demonstrate clinical improvement after 48 hours of IV therapy warrant repeat blood and urine cultures as well as imaging to evaluate for anatomic abnormalities or nephrolithiasis.[42]

A small subset of patients with pyelonephritis may be considered for outpatient therapy. These individuals must be less than 24 weeks pregnant, able to tolerate oral therapy, afebrile, and hemodynamically stable, with no chronic medical conditions or any history of preterm labor. Management includes a once-daily dose of ceftriaxone intramuscularly, followed by a 10-day regimen of oral cephalexin.[41]

Catheter-Associated Urinary Tract Infection

Antibiotic prophylaxis is not recommended for patients with short-term or long-term urinary catheters or those who intermittently catheterize themselves for prolonged periods of time.[32] Additionally, antibiotics should not be used prophylactically for catheter placement, removal, or catheter change. Urine cultures should be obtained from a newly placed catheter prior to initiating antimicrobial therapy in all catheterized patients who present with symptoms.[3]

Catheter-associated UTIs are often polymicrobial and more likely to be caused by multidrug-resistant organisms. Empirical therapy should be based on local resistance patterns and epidemiologic data regarding causative agents of catheter-associated UTIs.[43] Therefore, initial therapy with a fluoroquinolone or an aminoglycoside is reasonable, if local resistance data support their use.[32] Patients who exhibit a timely response to treatment should receive 7 days of antibiotics, whereas those with a delayed response require prolonged treatment of 10 days to 14 days.[32,43] Another important component of treatment involves replacement of or removal of the catheter if it has been in place greater than or equal to 2 weeks.[43]

Candida Urinary Tract Infection

Candiduria is associated with increased mortality rates, especially in ICU patients, if it reflects true infection of the urinary tract. A vast majority of patients with candiduria do not have UTIs due to *Candida*. The finding of yeast in the urine in previously healthy, asymptomatic patients should be verified with a second urine specimen. True infections are commonly caused by *C albicans*, which comprises 50% to 70% of isolates.[44]

C glabrata is another commonly isolated species and is more common in older adults and neonates, especially in the ICU setting.[44] Although most species of *Candida*, including *C albicans, C tropicalis*, and *C parapsilosis*, are successfully treated with fluconazole,[31] most strains of *C glabrata* are resistant to fluconazole.[44] *C krusei* is another fluconazole-resistant species but is uncommonly found in the urine.

For patients with persistent candiduria and a urinary catheter, removal of the catheter may suffice in clearing the infection,[31] but catheterized patients who are symptomatic should be treated with 14 days of fluconazole.[43] *Candida* in the urine of a critically ill patient should always be regarded as a potential sign of invasive candidiasis, regardless if urinary symptoms are present, and blood cultures as well as a retinal and skin examination should be performed.[31]

SUMMARY

UTIs are commonly encountered bacterial infections. Diagnosis of UTIs relies on the history and physical examination, evaluation of risk factors, and urinalysis results, all of which must be interpreted carefully. Urine cultures with susceptibility testing are not always necessary but should be performed during pregnancy, empirical treatment failure, and when an upper tract infection, complicated UTI, or recurrent UTI is suspected. *E coli* remains the most frequent cause of UTIs, but rising antimicrobial resistance has changed the landscape of empirical treatment. Practitioners must be familiar with local resistance patterns when prescribing and be able to distinguish UTIs from asymptomatic bacteriuria and candiduria to prevent further antimicrobial resistance.

REFERENCES

1. Barber AE, Norton JP, Spivak AM, et al. Urinary tract infections: current and emerging management strategies. Clin Infect Dis 2013;57(5):719–24.
2. Wang A, Nizran P, Malone MA, et al. Urinary tract infections. Prim Care 2013; 40(3):687–706.
3. Nicolle LE, Bradley S, Colgan R, et al. Infectious Diseases Society of America guidelines for the diagnosis and treatment of asymptomatic bacteriuria in adults. Clin Infect Dis 2005;40(5):643–54.
4. Gupta K, Hooton TM, Naber KG, et al. International clinical practice guidelines for the treatment of acute uncomplicated cystitis and pyelonephritis in women: a 2010 update by the Infectious Diseases Society of America and the European Society for Microbiology and Infectious Diseases. Clin Infect Dis 2011;52(5): e103–20.
5. Foxman B. Urinary tract infection syndromes: occurrence, recurrence, bacteriology, risk factors, and disease burden. Infect Dis Clin North Am 2014;28(1): 1–13.
6. Hooton TM. Clinical practice. Uncomplicated urinary tract infection. N Engl J Med 2012;366(11):1028–37.
7. Measley RE Jr, Levison ME. Host defense mechanisms in the pathogenesis of urinary tract infection. Med Clin North Am 1991;75(2):275–86.
8. Foxman B. Epidemiology of urinary tract infections: incidence, morbidity, and economic costs. Dis Mon 2003;49(2):53–70.
9. Raz R. Urinary tract infection in postmenopausal women. Korean J Urol 2011; 52(12):801–8.
10. Luthje P, Brauner H, Ramos NL, et al. Estrogen supports urothelial defense mechanisms. Sci Transl Med 2013;5(190):190ra80.

11. Hooton TM, Scholes D, Hughes JP, et al. A prospective study of risk factors for symptomatic urinary tract infection in young women. N Engl J Med 1996; 335(7):468–74.
12. Hooton TM, Hillier S, Johnson C, et al. Escherichia coli bacteriuria and contraceptive method. JAMA 1991;265(1):64–9.
13. Scholes D, Hooton TM, Roberts PL, et al. Risk factors for recurrent urinary tract infection in young women. J Infect Dis 2000;182(4):1177–82.
14. Russell DB, Roth NJ. Urinary tract infections in men in a primary care population. Aust Fam Physician 2001;30(2):177–9.
15. Ahmed AF, Solyman AA, Kamal SM. Potential host-related risk factors for recurrent urinary tract infection in Saudi women of childbearing age. Int Urogynecol J 2016;27(8):1245–53.
16. Mishra B, Srivastava R, Agarwal J, et al. Behavioral and psychosocial risk factors associated with first and recurrent cystitis in Indian women: A Case-control Study. Indian J Community Med 2016;41(1):27–33.
17. Badran YA, El-Kashef TA, Abdelaziz AS, et al. Impact of genital hygiene and sexual activity on urinary tract infection during pregnancy. Urol Ann 2015;7(4): 478–81.
18. Hooten T. Recurrent urinary tract infections in women. Int J Antimicrob Agents 2001;17(4):259–68.
19. Foxman B, Frerichs RR. Epidemiology of urinary tract infection: II. Diet, clothing, and urination habits. Am J Public Health 1985;75(11):1314–7.
20. Stapleton AE. Urinary tract infection in women: new pathogenic considerations. Curr Infect Dis Rep 2006;8(6):465–72.
21. Smith HS, Hughes JP, Hooton TM, et al. Antecedent antimicrobial use increases the risk of uncomplicated cystitis in young women. Clin Infect Dis 1997;25(1): 63–8.
22. Costelloe C, Metcalfe C, Lovering A, et al. Effect of antibiotic prescribing in primary care on antimicrobial resistance in individual patients: systematic review and meta-analysis. BMJ 2010;340:c2096.
23. Rivera-Sanchez R, Delgado-Ochoa D, Flores-Paz RR, et al. Prospective study of urinary tract infection surveillance after kidney transplantation. BMC Infect Dis 2010;10:245.
24. Byam PR, Pierre RB, Christie CD, et al. Antibiotic resistance among pathogens causing disease in Jamaican children with HIV/AIDS. West Indian Med J 2010; 59(4):386–92.
25. Richards MJ, Edwards JR, Culver DH, et al. Nosocomial infections in combined medical-surgical intensive care units in the United States. Infect Control Hosp Epidemiol 2000;21(8):510–5.
26. Haley RW, Hooton TM, Culver DH, et al. Nosocomial infections in U.S. hospitals, 1975-1976: estimated frequency by selected characteristics of patients. Am J Med 1981;70(4):947–59.
27. Classen DC, Larsen RA, Burke JP, et al. Prevention of catheter-associated bacteriuria: clinical trial of methods to block three known pathways of infection. Am J Infect Control 1991;19(3):136–42.
28. Tambyah PA, Halvorson KT, Maki DG. A prospective study of pathogenesis of catheter-associated urinary tract infections. Mayo Clin Proc 1999;74(2):131–6.
29. Clark KR, Higgs MJ. Urinary infection following out-patient flexible cystoscopy. Br J Urol 1990;66(5):503–5.
30. Lane DR, Takhar SS. Diagnosis and management of urinary tract infection and pyelonephritis. Emerg Med Clin North Am 2011;29(3):539–52.

31. Fisher JF. Candida urinary tract infections - epidemiology, pathogenesis, diagnosis, and treatment: executive summary. Clin Infect Dis 2011;52(Suppl 6): S429–32.
32. Hooton TM, Bradley SF, Cardenas DD, et al. Diagnosis, prevention, and treatment of catheter-associated urinary tract infection in adults: 2009 International Clinical Practice Guidelines from the Infectious Diseases Society of America. Clin Infect Dis 2010;50(5):625–63.
33. Deville WL, Yzermans JC, van Duijn NP, et al. The urine dipstick test useful to rule out infections. A meta-analysis of the accuracy. BMC Urol 2004;4:4.
34. Spoorenberg V, Prins JM, Opmeer BC, et al. The additional value of blood cultures in patients with complicated urinary tract infections. Clin Microbiol Infect 2014;20(8):O476–9.
35. ACR Appropriateness Criteria® in acute pyelonephritis. Agency for Healthcare Research and Quality. 2012. Available at: https://www.guideline.gov/summaries/summary/37923?. Accessed August 21, 2016.
36. Gupta K, Bhadelia N. Management of urinary tract infections from multidrug-resistant organisms. Infect Dis Clin North Am 2014;28(1):49–59.
37. Best practice policy statement on urologic surgery antimicrobial prophylaxis (2008). American Urological Association. 2008. Available at: http://www.auanet.org/education/guidelines/antimicrobial-prophylaxis.cfm. Accessed August 21, 2016.
38. FDA Drug Safety Administration: FDA updates warning for oral and injectable fluoroquinolone antibiotics due to disabling side effects. U.S. Food and Drug Administration. 2016. Available at: http://www.fda.gov/Drugs/DrugSafety/ucm511530.htm. Accessed August 21, 2016.
39. Grigoryan L, Trautner BW, Gupta K. Diagnosis and management of urinary tract infections in the outpatient setting: a review. JAMA 2014;312(16):1677–84.
40. Shepherd AK, Pottinger PS. Management of urinary tract infections in the era of increasing antimicrobial resistance. Med Clin North Am 2013;97(4):737–57, xii.
41. Jolley JA, Wing DA. Pyelonephritis in pregnancy: an update on treatment options for optimal outcomes. Drugs 2010;70(13):1643–55.
42. Matuszkiewicz-Rowinska J, Malyszko J, Wieliczko M. Urinary tract infections in pregnancy: old and new unresolved diagnostic and therapeutic problems. Arch Med Sci 2015;11(1):67–77.
43. Chenoweth CE, Gould CV, Saint S. Diagnosis, management, and prevention of catheter-associated urinary tract infections. Infect Dis Clin North Am 2014; 28(1):105–19.
44. Kauffman CA. Diagnosis and management of fungal urinary tract infection. Infect Dis Clin North Am 2014;28(1):61–74.

Sexually Transmitted Infections: A Medical Update

Patricia R. Jennings, PA-C, DrPH*, Ronald W. Flenner, MD

KEYWORDS

- STI • Genital infections • Syphilis • Gonorrhea • Chlamydia • Trichomonas

KEY POINTS

- After reading this article, the participant should be able to describe the current statistical trends of common sexually transmitted infections (STIs) in the United States.
- After reading this article, the participant should be able to discuss the current screening and diagnostic testing available for common STIs in the United States.
- After reading this article, the participant should be able to incorporate the current treatment plan available for common STIs in the United States into their practice.
- After reading this article, the participant should be able to discuss prevention strategies for common STIs in the United States.

The term sexually transmitted infections (STIs) refers to a variety of clinical syndromes and infections caused by pathogens that can be acquired and transmitted through sexual activity. The Centers for Disease Control and Prevention (CDC) estimates that nearly 20 million new STIs occur every year in this country, half among young people aged 15 to 24, and account for almost $16 billion in health care costs. Many STIs are undiagnosed and others are not reportable to the CDC (herpes, trichomonas, human papilloma virus), therefore the actual number may be much higher. In addition to increasing a person's risk for acquiring and transmitting human immunodeficiency virus (HIV) infection, STIs can lead to severe reproductive health complications, such as infertility and ectopic pregnancy.[1] Physician assistants (PAs) play a critical role in identifying, treating, and preventing STIs. As part of the clinical encounter, PAs should routinely obtain sexual histories from their patients and address risk reduction.

Several factors contribute to the spread of STIs, including biologic, social, economic, and behavioral. STIs are acquired during unprotected sex with an infected

Disclosure: (P.R. Jennings) Faculty member of the CDC-sponsored National Network of Sexually Transmitted Disease Clinical Prevention Training Centers.
Eastern Virginia Medical School, 700 West Onley Road, Norfolk, VA 23507, USA
* Corresponding author.
E-mail address: jenninpa@evms.edu

Physician Assist Clin 2 (2017) 207–218
http://dx.doi.org/10.1016/j.cpha.2016.12.004   physicianassistant.theclinics.com
2405-7991/17/Published by Elsevier Inc.

partner. Unfortunately, many STIs either do not produce any signs or symptoms or the signs and symptoms are so mild that they are unnoticed. Therefore, many infected individuals do not know that they need treatment and may unintentionally transmit their infection to an uninfected partner. Certain racial and ethnic groups have high rates of STIs when compared with white individuals.[2] STIs disproportionately affect disadvantaged people and people in social networks in which high-risk sexual behavior is common. Many studies document the association of substance abuse with STIs and the introduction of new illicit substances into communities can alter sexual behavior in high-risk sexual networks.[3] Another important factor contributing to the spread of STIs in the United States is the stigma associated with STIs and the general discomfort of eliciting a sexual history from patients of all ages. An innovative communication strategy that normalizes perceptions of sexual health and STI prevention may be helpful in identifying high-risk behaviors, infected individuals, and prevention strategies.

This article reviews recent demographics, as well as current screening, diagnostic testing, and treatment of syphilis, herpes, gonorrhea, chlamydia, trichomonas, and nongonococcal urethritis.

SYPHILIS
Overview

Syphilis has been called "the great imitator" because it has so many possible symptoms, many of which look like symptoms from other diseases. The painless ulcer can be confused for an ingrown hair, zipper cut, or a seemingly harmless bump. The nonpruritic body rash that develops during the secondary stage of syphilis can show up on the palms of the hands and soles of the feet, all over the body, or in just a few places. Approximately 20,000 cases of syphilis were reported to the CDC in 2014 compared with 6103 cases in 2001. Before 2013, increasing syphilis rates were mainly due to cases in men, particularly in men who have sex with men (MSM). But from 2013 to 2014, syphilis case rates increased 22.7% in women and the congenital syphilis case rate increased 37% (from 2012 to 2014).[4]

Syphilis is caused by the spirochete *Treponema pallidum*. Syphilis is transmissible by sexual contact with infectious lesions, from mother to fetus in utero, and via blood product transfusion. If untreated, it progresses through 4 stages: primary, secondary, latent, and tertiary. Primary syphilis is characterized by the development of a painless chancre at the site of transmission after an incubation period of 3 to 6 weeks. The lesion has a punched-out base and rolled edges and is highly infectious (Fig. 1). Secondary syphilis develops approximately 4 to 10 weeks after the appearance of the primary lesion. During this stage, the spirochetes multiply and spread throughout the body. Secondary syphilis lesions are quite variable in their manifestations. Systemic manifestations include malaise, fever, myalgias, arthralgias, lymphadenopathy, and rash. Latent syphilis is a stage at which the features of secondary syphilis have resolved, although patients remain seroreactive. Latent syphilis acquired within the preceding year is referred to as early latent syphilis; all other cases of latent syphilis are late latent syphilis or syphilis of unknown duration.[1] Approximately one-third of patients with untreated latent syphilis go on to develop tertiary syphilis, whereas the rest remain asymptomatic. Currently, tertiary syphilis disease is rare.[5] *T pallidum* can infect the central nervous system and result in neurosyphilis, which can occur at any stage of syphilis. Early neurologic clinical manifestations (ie, cranial nerve dysfunction, meningitis, stroke, acute altered mental status, and auditory or ophthalmic abnormalities) are usually present within the first few months or years of infection.

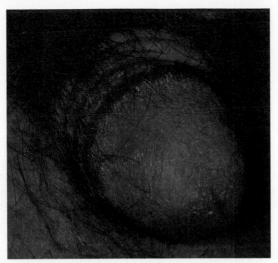

Fig. 1. Syphilis lesion with a punched-out base and rolled edges.

Diagnostic Considerations

Darkfield examinations and tests to detect *T pallidum* directly from lesion exudate or tissue are the definitive methods for diagnosing early syphilis. A presumptive diagnosis of syphilis requires the use of 2 tests: a nontreponemal test (ie, Venereal Disease Research Laboratory [VDRL] or Rapid Plasma Reagin [RPR]) and a treponemal test (ie, fluorescent treponemal antibody absorbed [FTA-ABS] tests, the *T pallidum* passive particle agglutination [TP-PA] assay, various enzyme immunoassays [EIAs], treponemal chemoluminescence test [CIA], or rapid treponemal assay).[1] There are only a few treponemal-based tests approved by the Food and Drug Administration (FDA) that are commercially available in the United States. The use of only one type of serologic test is insufficient for the diagnosis of syphilis.

Nontreponemal test antibody titers are used to follow treatment response and results should be reported quantitatively. A fourfold change in titer is considered necessary to demonstrate a clinically significant difference between 2 nontreponemal test results (for example, before and after treatment) using the SAME serologic test method (Fig. 2). Although the VDRL and RPR are valid assays, results from the 2 tests cannot be compared directly. Some clinical laboratories are using a reverse screening algorithm for syphilis testing (Fig. 3). Reverse screening begins with a treponemal test, and if positive then a nontreponemal test with titer is performed to guide patient management. However, the CDC recommends the use of the RPR-based screening algorithm. When there is a low epidemiologic risk or clinical probability of syphilis, the positive predictive value of an isolated unconfirmed reactive treponemal CIA test or EIA is low.

According to the 2015 CDC sexually transmitted disease treatment guidelines, pregnant women who are seropositive for syphilis should be considered infected unless there is evidence of adequate treatment in the medical records. Serologic titers should be checked monthly if the patient is at risk for reinfection. Per CDC guidelines, any woman who delivers a stillborn infant after 20 weeks' gestation also should be tested for syphilis.[1]

The diagnosis of neurosyphilis depends on a combination of cerebrospinal fluid (CSF) tests (CSF cell count or protein and a reactive CSF-VDRL) in the presence of reactive serologic test results and neurologic signs and symptoms.[1] Of note, a

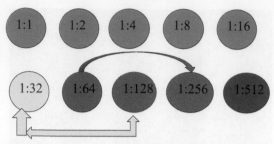

Fig. 2. A fourfold change in titer is considered necessary to demonstrate a clinically significant difference between 2 nontreponemal test results (for example, before and after treatment) using the SAME serologic test method. Initial Patient Titer = 1:128. 3 months after treatment titer = 1:32. 1:32 represents a fourfold dilution decrease from 1:128. A titer of 1:64, 1:128 or 1:256 is not significant. A titer of 1:512 represents a fourfold increase from 1:128.

CSF-RPR is *not used* because of the high false-negative rate when compared with the CSF-VDRL. Follow-up testing for patients with a positive CSF-VDRL is with the VDRL (either repeat CSF-VDRL or serum VDRL).

Treatment

Parenteral benzathine penicillin G (Bicillin L-A) is the treatment of choice to achieve clinical resolution of primary and secondary syphilis. Selection of the appropriate

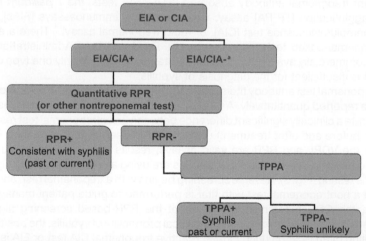

Fig. 3. CDC-recommended algorithm for reverse-sequence syphilis screening. EIAs – some detect both IGG and IGM. CIA, chemiluminescence assay. Recent change to recommendation from treponemal test using a different platform to TPPA. Based on published sensitivity and specificity data, the TPPA is currently considered the most suitable confirmatory test. FTA-ABS with lower specificity than other treponemal tests and probably lower sensitivity. FTA-ABS requires trained personnel and a decidated flourescence microscope. [a] If incubating or primary syphilis is suspected, treat with benzathine PCN 2.4 million units single dose. (*Adapted from* Centers for Disease Control and Prevention (CDC). Discordant results from reverse sequence syphilis screening–five laboratories, United States, 2006–2010. MMWR Morb Mortal Wkly Rep 2011;60(5):133–7.)

penicillin preparation is important, because *T pallidum* can reside in sequestered sites (eg, the central nervous system and aqueous humor) that are poorly accessed by some forms of penicillin. Combinations of benzathine-procaine penicillin (Bicillin C-R), and oral penicillin preparations are not considered appropriate for the treatment of syphilis. The recommended regimen for adults with primary, secondary, or early latent syphilis is benzathine penicillin G 2.4 million units intramuscularly (IM) in a single dose (usually split into 2 injections of 1.2 million units each, one in the right and one in the left gluteal muscle within minutes of each other). The treatment of late latent syphilis or syphilis of unknown duration is benzathine penicillin G 7.2 million units total, administered as 3 doses of 2.4 million units IM each at 1-week intervals.[1]

Pregnant women with primary or secondary syphilis who are allergic to penicillin should be desensitized and treated with penicillin.[1] In nonpregnant, penicillin-allergic persons who have primary or secondary syphilis, regimens of doxycycline and tetracycline have been used for many years. Limited clinical studies have been conducted with other regimens; however, optimal dose and duration of therapy along with resistance and treatment failures suggest that they should not be used as first-line treatment for syphilis in patients who are allergic to penicillin.[1] It is best to consult an infectious disease specialist for treatment of syphilis in a patients who is allergic to penicillin who cannot tolerate doxycycline or tetracycline and in individuals infected with HIV. All patients, regardless of treatment regimen, should be followed closely after treatment with documentation of a decrease in nontreponemal titers.

Management of Sex Partners

Persons who have had sexual contact with a person who receives a diagnosis of primary, secondary, or early latent syphilis within 90 days preceding the diagnosis should be treated presumptively for early syphilis, even if serologic test results are negative.

Prevention

Prevention counseling is most effective if provided in a nonjudgmental and empathetic manner appropriate to the patient's culture, language, gender, sexual orientation, age, and developmental level. Prevention counseling for STIs should be offered to all sexually active adolescents and to all adults who have received an STI diagnosis, have had an STI in the past year, or have multiple sexual partners.

HERPES
Overview

Genital herpes is a common, chronic, lifelong viral infection caused by herpes simplex virus type 1 (HSV-1) or herpes simplex virus type 2 (HSV-2). Most people are infected with HSV-1 during childhood from nonsexual contact. More than half of the population in the United States has antibodies to HSV-1, even if they do not show any signs or symptoms. HSV-1 also can be spread from the mouth to the genitals through oral sex. This is why an increasing proportion of anogenital infections have been attributed to HSV-1, which is especially prominent among young women and MSM. HSV-2 infection is more common among women than among men. Infection is more easily transmitted from men to women than from women to men. Most cases of recurrent genital herpes are caused by HSV-2. Most individuals infected with HSV-2 are unaware that they are infected and, consequently, most genital herpes infections are transmitted by persons unaware that they have the infection or are asymptomatic when the transmission occurs. The CDC suggests that the management of genital HSV should address the chronic nature of the infection rather than focusing on the treatment of acute episodes.[1]

Diagnostic Considerations

The classic lesions of genital herpes often resemble small pimples or blisters that eventually crust over and finally scab like a small cut. These lesions may take anywhere from 2 to 4 weeks to heal fully. During this time, some people will experience a second crop of lesions, and some will experience flulike symptoms, including fever and swollen glands, particularly in the lymph nodes near the groin. Headache and painful urination also sometimes accompany full-blown symptoms of first episodes.

The clinical diagnosis of genital herpes can be difficult and the sensitivity of a viral culture is low, especially for recurrent lesions. Failure to detect HSV by culture does not indicate an absence of HSV infection, because viral shedding is intermittent. Tzanck preparation is an insensitive and nonspecific method of diagnosing genital lesions and therefore should not be relied on.[1]

The type of HSV infection affects prognosis and subsequent counseling; therefore, type-specific testing to distinguish HSV-1 from HSV-2 is recommended. Both type-specific and type-common antibodies to HSV develop during the first several weeks after infection and persist indefinitely in an immunocompetent individual. The sensitivities of glycoprotein G type-specific tests for the detection of HSV-2 antibody vary from 80% to 98%.[1] Because most HSV-2 infections are sexually acquired, the presence of type-specific HSV-2 antibodies implies anogenital infection. Accurate type-specific HSV serologic assays are based on the HSV-specific glycoprotein G2 (HSV-2) and glycoprotein G1 (HSV-1). Providers should request type-specific glycoprotein G (gG)-based serologic assays only when serology is performed for their patients.[6] Due to commonly shared antigens, infections with one type of HSV, in the presence of antibody to the other type, may produce an amnestic response with the level of the preexisting antibody becoming higher than the antibody titer of the current infection. Definitive diagnosis of HSV type should be made by polymerase chain reaction (PCR).[7]

PCR has been the diagnostic standard method for HSV infections of the central nervous system and viral culture has been the test of choice for HSV genital infection. However, HSV PCR, with its consistently and substantially higher rate of HSV detection, could replace viral culture as the gold standard for the diagnosis of genital herpes in people with active mucocutaneous lesions, regardless of anatomic location or viral type.

Treatment

Management with antiviral therapy provides clinical benefit to most symptomatic individuals. Dosing information can be found in the CDC Sexually Transmitted Disease Guidelines, 2015.[1] Systemic antiviral medications (acyclovir, famciclovir, valacyclovir) can partially control the signs and symptoms of genital herpes; however, these drugs neither eradicate latent virus nor affect the risk, frequency, or severity of recurrences after the drug is discontinued.[1] Topical therapy with antiviral drugs offers minimal clinical benefit and is discouraged.

Prevention

Education and counseling of infected individuals and their sex partners regarding the lifelong nature of the infection and the possibility of sexual as well as perinatal transmission should be provided along with methods to reduce transmission.

GONORRHEA
Overview

Gonorrhea is the second most commonly reported notifiable disease in the United States. It can cause infections in the genitals, rectum, and throat. Infections due to *Neisseria gonorrhoeae*, like those resulting from *Chlamydia trachomatis*, are a major cause of pelvic inflammatory disease (PID) in the United States. PID can lead to serious outcomes in women, such as tubal infertility, ectopic pregnancy, and chronic pelvic pain. In addition, epidemiologic and biologic studies provide evidence that gonococcal and chlamydial infections facilitate the transmission of HIV infection. The rate of gonorrhea increased 5.1% since 2013, and increased 10.5% since 2010. As was observed in 2013, in 2014 the rate of reported gonorrhea cases among men (120.1 cases per 100,000 men) was higher than the rate among women (101.3 cases per 100,000 women).[4]

Urethral infections caused by *N gonorrhoeae* among men are usually symptomatic; however, infections in women are often asymptomatic until complications such as PID have occurred. The asymptomatic nature and harmful sequelae in women has prompted the CDC to recommend annual screening for *N gonorrhoeae* and *C trachomatis* in all sexually active women younger than 25 years. Additional risk factors for gonorrhea include inconsistent condom use among persons who are not in mutually monogamous relationships, previous or coexisting STIs, and exchanging sex for money or drugs.[1]

Diagnostic Considerations

Culture and nucleic acid amplification test (NAAT) are available for the detection of genitourinary infection with *N gonorrhoeae*. NAAT allows for the widest variety of FDA-cleared specimen types, including endocervical swabs, vaginal swabs, urethral swabs (men), and urine (both men and women). Culture is available for detection of rectal, oropharyngeal, and conjunctival infections. Some laboratories have met clinical laboratory improvement amendment (CLIA) regulatory requirements and established performance specifications for using NAAT with rectal and oropharyngeal swab specimens. You should consult your laboratory vendor before ordering NAAT from those sites. In cases of suspected or documented treatment failure, clinicians should perform both culture and antimicrobial susceptibility testing because nonculture tests cannot provide antimicrobial susceptibility results.

Treatment

N gonorrhoeae has progressively developed resistance to each of the antimicrobials used for treatment of gonorrhea. Most recently, declining susceptibility to cefixime resulted in a change to the CDC treatment guidelines, so that dual therapy with ceftriaxone (250 mg IM) and azithromycin (1 g by mouth) is now the only CDC-recommended treatment regimen for gonorrhea. To maximize adherence with recommended therapies, medication for gonococcal infection should be provided on site and directly observed.

A test-of-cure is not needed for persons who receive a diagnosis of uncomplicated urogenital or rectal gonorrhea who are treated with any of the recommended or alternative regimens. However, any person with pharyngeal gonorrhea who is treated with an alternative regimen should be retested more than 14 days after treatment.[1]

Management of Sex Partners

Persons having sexual contact with the infected individual within the 60 days preceding the onset of symptoms, should be evaluated, tested, and given presumptive dual treatment. To minimize transmission, persons treated for gonorrhea should be instructed to abstain from sexual activity for 7 days after their treatment as well as 7 days after their sex partner was treated. All persons who receive a diagnosis of gonorrhea should be tested for other STIs, including chlamydia, syphilis, and HIV.

Expedited partner therapy (EPT), also termed patient-delivered partner therapy (PDPT), is the clinical practice of treating the sex partners of persons who receive chlamydia or gonorrhea diagnoses by providing medications or prescriptions to the patient. Patients then provide partners with these therapies without the health care provider having examined the partner. EPT is legal in most states; however, providers should visit http://www.cdc.gov/std/ept to obtain updated information for their state. Providing patients with appropriately packaged medication is the preferred approach to EPT/PDPT because data on the efficacy of EPT/PDPT using prescriptions are limited and many persons do not fill the prescriptions given to them by a sex partner.[1]

CHLAMYDIA
Overview

Chlamydia, caused by infection with C trachomatis, is the most common notifiable disease in the United States. It is among the most prevalent of all STIs, and since 1994, has comprised the largest proportion of all STIs reported to the CDC. Chlamydial infections in women are usually asymptomatic; however, untreated infection can result in PID, which is a major cause of infertility, ectopic pregnancy, and chronic pelvic pain. Epidemiologic and biologic studies provide evidence that gonococcal and chlamydial infections facilitate the transmission of HIV infection. Approximately 1.5 million cases of chlamydia were reported to the CDC in 2014, representing an overall 2.8% increase. The reported case rate among women was approximately 2 times the case rate among men in 2014, likely reflecting a larger number of women screened for this infection. The lower rate among men also suggests that many of the sex partners of women with chlamydia are not receiving a diagnosis of chlamydia or being reported as having chlamydia.[4] All sexually active women younger than 25 years should be screened for chlamydia at least once per year.

Diagnostic Considerations

Optimal urogenital specimen types for chlamydia screening using NAAT include first-catch urine (men) and vaginal swabs (women). C trachomatis infections can be diagnosed in women by testing first-catch urine or collecting swab specimens from the endocervix or vagina. NAAT in men includes collection of urethral swab specimens or first-catch urine specimens. NAAT first-catch urine specimens in women have higher false-negative results when compared with first-catch urine specimens in men. It is difficult to test for rectal and oropharyngeal C trachomatis infections in persons engaging in receptive anal or oral intercourse because NAATs are not FDA-cleared for such use. However, research has demonstrated that NAATs have improved sensitivity and specificity compared with culture for detection of C trachomatis at rectal sites and oropharyngeal sites among men.

Treatment

The CDC-recommended regimen for uncomplicated urogenital infections is azithromycin 1 g orally in a single dose or doxycycline 100 mg orally twice a day for 7 days. A meta-analysis of 12 randomized clinical trials of azithromycin versus doxycycline for the treatment of urogenital chlamydial infection demonstrated that the treatments were equally efficacious, with microbial cure rates of 97% and 98%, respectively.[1]

Test-of-cure to detect therapeutic failure is not advised for persons treated with the recommended or alternative regimens unless therapeutic adherence is in question, symptoms persist, or reinfection is suspected. If a test-of-cure is performed, it must be done more than 3 weeks after completion of therapy, as the continued presence of nonviable organisms can lead to false-positive results.[1]

Special Considerations

In pregnancy, a test-of-cure to document chlamydial eradication (preferably by NAAT) 3 to 4 weeks after completion of therapy is recommended because severe sequelae can occur in mothers and neonates if the infection persists. In addition, all pregnant women who have chlamydial infection diagnosed should be retested 3 months after treatment.

Women younger than 25 years and those at increased risk for chlamydia should be rescreened during the third trimester to prevent maternal postnatal complications and chlamydial infection in the infant.[1]

Management of Sex Partners

Persons having sexual contact with the infected individual within the 60 days preceding the onset of symptoms should be evaluated, tested, and given presumptive treatment. To minimize transmission, persons treated for chlamydia should be instructed to abstain from sexual activity for 7 days after their treatment, as well as 7 days after their sex partner was treated. All persons who receive a diagnosis of chlamydia should be tested for other STIs, including, syphilis, and HIV.

EPT, also termed PDPT, is the clinical practice of treating the sex partners of persons who receive chlamydia or gonorrhea diagnoses by providing medications or prescriptions to the patient. Patients then provide partners with these therapies without the health care provider having examined the partner. EPT is legal in most states. However, providers should visit http://www.cdc.gov/std/ept to obtain updated information for their state. Providing patients with appropriately packaged medication is the preferred approach to EPT/PDPT because data on the efficacy of EPT/PDPT using prescriptions are limited and many persons do not fill the prescriptions given to them by a sex partner.[1]

NONGONOCOCCAL URETHRITIS
Overview

Urethritis, as characterized by urethral inflammation, can result from infectious and noninfectious conditions. Symptoms, if present, include dysuria; urethral pruritis; and mucoid, mucopurulent, or purulent discharge. Signs of urethral discharge on examination also can be present in persons without symptoms. Nongonococcal urethritis (NGU) is an infection of the urethra caused by pathogens other than gonorrhea. Several kinds of pathogens can cause NGU, including *C trachomatis, Ureaplasma urealyticum, Trichomonas vaginalis*, HSV, *Haemophilus* vaginalis, and *Mycoplasma genitalium. M genitalium,* which can be sexually transmitted, is associated with symptoms of urethritis as well as urethral inflammation and accounts for 15% to 25% of NGU cases in the United States. Unfortunately, there is no FDA-cleared diagnostic test for *M genitalium*.

Diagnostic Considerations

NGU is a nonspecific diagnosis that can have many infectious etiologies. NGU is confirmed in symptomatic men when staining of urethral secretions indicates inflammation without gram-negative diplococci. Clinicians should attempt to obtain objective evidence of urethral inflammation. However, if point-of-care diagnostic tests are not available (eg, Gram, methylene blue, or gentian violet stain microscopy), all men should be tested by NAAT and treated with drug regimens effective against both gonorrhea and chlamydia. All men who have confirmed NGU should be tested for chlamydia and gonorrhea. Testing for *T vaginalis* should be considered in areas or populations of high prevalence.

Treatment

Presumptive treatment should be initiated at the time of NGU diagnosis. Azithromycin and doxycycline are highly effective for chlamydial urethritis. NGU associated with *M genitalium* currently responds better to azithromycin than doxycycline. A directly observed, single-dose treatment regimen may be associated with higher rates of compliance over other regimens. Men treated for NGU should be instructed to abstain from sexual intercourse until they and their partner(s) have been adequately treated. Men who receive a diagnosis of NGU should be tested for HIV and syphilis.

Persistent Nongonococcal Urethritis

The value of extended antimicrobial therapy in men who have persistent symptoms after treatment for NGU has not been demonstrated. Men who did not comply with the initial treatment regimen or were reexposed to an untreated sex partner should be retreated. Recent studies have shown that the most common cause of persistent or recurrent NGU is *M genitalium.* If doxycycline was given as the initial treatment regimen, azithromycin 1 g orally in a single dose should be administered. *T vaginalis* is another possibility, and although no NAAT for *T vaginalis* has been FDA-cleared for men, several large reference laboratories have performed the necessary CLIA validation of urine-based *T vaginalis* NAAT for men. In areas in which *T vaginalis* is prevalent, men who have sex with women and have persistent or recurrent NGU should be presumptively treated with metronidazole 2 g orally in a single dose or tinidazole 2 g orally in a single dose.[1]

Management of Sex Partners

All partners of men with NGU within the preceding 60 days should be referred for evaluation, testing, and presumptive treatment with a drug regimen effective against chlamydia.[1] To avoid reinfection, sex partners should abstain from sexual intercourse until they and their partner(s) are adequately treated.

TRICHOMONIASIS
Overview

Trichomoniasis, caused by *T vaginalis,* is the most prevalent nonviral STI in the United States, affecting an estimated 3.7 million persons.[1] Some infected men have symptoms of urethritis, epididymitis, or prostatitis. Some infected women have vaginal discharge that might be diffuse, malodorous, or yellow-green with or without vulvar irritation. However, most individuals are asymptomatic and untreated infections might last for months to years.[1] It is important to identify and treat *T vaginalis* infection, as it is associated with twofold to threefold risk for HIV acquisition, preterm birth, and other adverse pregnancy outcomes among pregnant women.[1]

Diagnostic Considerations

The use of NAAT, a highly sensitive and specific test for *T vaginalis*, is recommended. NAAT often detects 3 to 5 times more *T vaginalis* infections than wet-mount microscopy. The APTIMA *T vaginalis* assay and the BD Probe Tec TV Qx Amplified DNA Assay are FDA-cleared assays for detection of *T vaginalis* from vaginal, endocervical, or urine specimens from women. Other FDA-cleared tests to detect *T vaginalis* in vaginal secretions include OSOM Trichomonas Rapid Test and the Affirm VP III.[1] Because of cost and availability, the most common method for detection of *T vaginalis* in women is a microscopic evaluation of wet preparations of genital secretions. Unfortunately, the sensitivity of wet mount is low in vaginal specimens and even lower in men (urethral specimens, urine sediment, and semen). Therefore, treatment may be based on signs/symptoms.

Treatment

Treatment reduces the signs and symptoms of *T vaginalis* infection. The recommended regimen is metronidazole 2 g orally in a single dose or tinidazole 2 g orally in a single dose. The nitroimidazoles are the only class of antimicrobial medications known to be effective against *T vaginalis* infections. Alcohol consumption should be avoided during treatment and abstinence should continue for 24 hours after metronidazole or 72 hours after tinidazole to avoid the possibility of a disulfiramlike reaction. Although tinidazole is generally more expensive, it reaches higher levels in serum and the genitourinary tract, has a longer half-life, and has fewer side effects when compared with metronidazole. Metronidazole gel does not reach therapeutic levels in the urethra and perivaginal glands and therefore it is not recommended.[1]

Persistent or Recurrent Trichomoniasis

Although most recurrent *T vaginalis* infections are due to reinfection, some infections might be attributed to antimicrobial resistance (metronidazole 4%–10%; tinidazole 1%). Single-dose therapy should be avoided to treat recurrent trichomoniasis and a regimen of metronidazole 500 mg orally twice daily for 7 days is recommended.[1]

Pregnancy

T vaginalis infection in pregnant women is associated with adverse pregnancy outcomes, particularly premature rupture of membranes, preterm delivery, and delivery of a low-birthweight infant.[1] Although metronidazole crosses the placenta, data suggest that it poses a low risk to pregnant women. No evidence of teratogenicity or mutagenic effects in infants has been found in multiple cross-sectional and cohort studies. Women can be treated with 2 g metronidazole orally in a single dose at any stage of pregnancy.[1]

Human Immunodeficiency Virus Infection

Up to 53% of women with HIV infection also are infected with *T vaginalis*. *T vaginalis* infection in these women is significantly associated with PID and treatment of trichomoniasis is associated with significant decreases in genital-tract HIV viral load and viral shedding.[1] The recommended treatment regimen for women with HIV infection who are found to be infected with *T vaginalis* is metronidazole 500 mg orally twice daily for 7 days. Retesting is recommended within 3 months following initial treatment, and NAAT is encouraged because of higher sensitivity of these tests.[1]

Management of Sexual Partners

Concurrent treatment of all sex partners is critical for symptomatic relief, microbiologic cure, and prevention of transmission.[1] To avoid reinfection, patients should abstain from sexual intercourse until they and their partner(s) are adequately treated.

SUMMARY

The term STI refers to a variety of clinical syndromes and infections caused by pathogens that can be acquired and transmitted through sexual activity. The CDC estimates that nearly 20 million new STIs occur every year in this country and account for almost $16 billion in health care costs. In addition to increasing a person's risk for acquiring and transmitting HIV infection, STIs can lead to severe reproductive health complications, such as infertility and ectopic pregnancy. Many STIs are undiagnosed and others are not reportable to the CDC (herpes, trichomonas, human papilloma virus), therefore the actual number may be much higher. PAs play a critical role in identifying, treating, and preventing STIs. As part of the clinical encounter, PAs should routinely obtain sexual histories from their patients and address risk reduction.

REFERENCES

1. CDC. Sexually transmitted diseases treatment guidelines. MMWR Recomm Rep 2015;64:1–137.
2. Chandra A. Impaired fecundity in the United States: 1982-1995. Fam Plann Perspect 1998;30:34–42.
3. Beltrami J, Wright-DeAguero L, Fullilove M, et al. Substance abuse and the spread of sexually transmitted diseases. Commissioned paper for the IOM Committee on Prevention and Control of STDs. 1997.
4. CDC. 2014 sexually transmitted disease surveillance. Retrieved from CDC. Available at: http://www.cdc.gov/std/stats14/gonorrhea.htm. Accessed August 18, 2016.
5. Chandrasekar P. Syphilis. Medscape website. 2016. Available at: http://emedicine.medscape.com/article/229461-overview#a3. Accessed August 18, 2016.
6. LeGrolf J, Pere H, Belec L. Diagnosis of genital herpes simplex virus infection in the clinical laboratory. Virol J 2014;11:83.
7. Interpretive Handbook Test 87998: Herpes Simplex Virus (HSV) Antibody Screen, IgM, by EIA, Serum. Available at: http://www.mayomedicallaboratories.com/interpretive-guide/?alpha=H&unit_code=87998. Accessed August 18, 2016.

An Overview of Best Practice Guidelines for *Mycobacterium tuberculosis* Screening and Treatment

Nancy Ivansek, PA-C, MA[a,b],*

KEYWORDS

- Active TB • Latent TB (LTBI) • Mantoux tuberculin skin test (TST)
- Interferon gamma release assay (IGRA) • Purified protein derivative (PPD)
- *Mycobacterium tuberculosis*

KEY POINTS

- For the tuberculosis (TB) elimination goal to be reached in the United States, screening for latent TB and active TB must be used and focused on high-risk populations, such as the homeless, immigrants from endemic areas, and prisoners.
- The appropriate choice of a screening test (TST vs IGRA) for latent TB takes into consideration the age of the patient, likelihood of returning for follow-up visits, cost of the test, and any underlying comorbidities.
- Treatment of latent TB is important in reducing the potential pool of convertors to active TB disease.
- Treatment of active TB disease is most successful when attention is paid to the number of doses of medication the patient receives and when it is administered following direct observation technique.

INTRODUCTION

In 2014, the Centers for Disease Control and Prevention (CDC) estimated an incidence rate for new tuberculosis (TB) cases reported in the United States to be 3.0 cases per 100,000 persons.[1] Although the number of cases of TB had declined from 2013 to 2014, the rate of decline was the smallest decrease in more than a decade.[1] The elimination goal of less than 1 case per 1 million persons was set in 1989 and reaffirmed in 1999. The present incidence rate has prompted the CDC to call for vigilant surveillance

The author has nothing to disclose.
[a] Clinical Curriculum, Physician Assistant Program, Case Western Reserve University, Cleveland, OH, USA; [b] Infectious Disease Department, Cleveland and Clinic Foundation, Cleveland, OH, USA
* 8735 Jamesway Court, Mentor, OH 44060.
E-mail address: nxi49@case.edu

Physician Assist Clin 2 (2017) 219–227
http://dx.doi.org/10.1016/j.cpha.2016.12.005   **physicianassistant.theclinics.com**

and active prevention measures, including screening and treating both latent tuberculosis infection (LTBI) and active TB.[1]

LATENT VERSUS ACTIVE DISEASE

Tuberculosis is caused by a group of 5 related species that form the *Mycobacterium tuberculosis* complex: *Mycobacterium bovis, Mycobacterium microti, Mycobacterium africanum, Mycobacterium canettii*, and *M tuberculosis*. In the United States, most TB cases are caused by *M tuberculosis*. In 1882, Dr Robert Koch discovered the TB bacillus.[1] A characteristic of *M tuberculosis* is the tendency to form dense clusters of bacilli. A defining characteristic of the bacilli in this genus is acid-fastness; the ability to withstand decolorization with acid-alcohol rinse after staining with carbolfuchsin or auramine-rhodamine. Because of this characteristic, *Mycobacterium* are referred to as acid-fast bacilli or AFB.[2] Mycobacterium are obligate aerobes, intercellular pathogens with slow growth rates. They are known to form granulomatous reactions in a normal host. TB transmission occurs almost exclusively from human to human. Most cases are acquired from individuals with acid-fast–positive sputum. Approximately 17% of cases can be spread by individuals with AFB-negative sputum.[2]

Most individuals exposed to *M tuberculosis* contain the illness and never acquire active disease.[2] They will have a positive tuberculin skin test (TST) or interferon gamma release assay (IGRA) test, and are normally found to have a normal chest radiograph and sputum testing that is negative. TB in the body is present but inactive. This is known as latent disease.[3] Latent TB infection (LTBI) is not communicable, and patients are asymptomatic. Most cases of active disease are communicable. The definition of active disease includes symptoms of a cough for 3 or more weeks, hemoptysis, night sweats, unexplained weight loss, and extreme fatigue. The lifetime risk for someone with latent disease developing active disease ranges between 5% and 10%. The risk is inversely proportional to age at the time of infection, thus children with latent disease are at greater risk than older adults with latent infection of developing active TB. Those individuals who have LTBI and medical comorbidities, especially immuno-compromising conditions such as human immunodeficiency virus (HIV) infection, recent bone marrow transplantation, or a malignant neoplasm, are also at increased risk of developing active disease.[3]

SCREENING TESTS

Before 2001, the TST was the only commercially available immunologic test approved in the United States for the screening of *M tuberculosis*. The IGRA was developed in response to some of the recognized problems of administration and reading the TST. The TST requires appropriate intradermal administration by the Mantoux method of 0.1 mL of purified protein tuberculin derivative (PPD). The injection is placed on the volar surface of the forearm. When correctly placed, the injection should produce a wheal 6 to 10 mm in diameter.[3] For the most accurate results, the patient must return to have the test read in 48 to 72 hours by an experienced health care worker (Fig. 1).[4] Test results can be influenced by previous vaccination of Bacille Calmette-Guerin (BCG) and previous exposure to nontuberculous mycobacterium.[5]

In 2001, the Quantiferon-TB test (QFT) became the first IGRA approved by the Food and Drug Administration (FDA) as an adjunct test to be used in the diagnosis of TB. The specificity of the QFT proved to be less than the TST, and in 2005, the test was taken off the market but other IGRA tests were developed that had improved specificity.[5] The CDC issued guidelines for the use of IGRAs initially in 2003.[5] As new IGRA testing became available, the CDC guidelines were updated, with the latest updates being

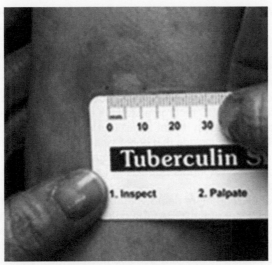

Fig. 1. Measurement of TST at 48 hours. (*From* Centers for Disease Control and Prevention. Testing for TB infection. Available at: http://www.cdc.gov/tb/topic/testing/tbtest types.htm. Accessed August 17, 2016)

released in 2010.[5] Two IGRA tests are available in many countries, including the United States: the Quantiferon-TB Gold in Tube (QFT-GIT) and the T-Spot TB assay. In 2015, the Quantiferon-TB Gold Plus (QFT-Plus) became available for use in Europe but is not available in North America.[5]

Neither the TST nor IGRA can determine if an individual has active or latent disease and cannot be used as a single tool to make this distinction. Neither test should be used to monitor treatment or therapy outcome. Determining what test should be used to screen for *M tuberculosis* depends on the reasons for testing, the context of the testing, test availability, and the cost-effectiveness of the test. Review of studies comparing sensitivity, specificity, and test agreement between the TST and IGRA vary with respect to which test is better.[5]

RECOMMENDATIONS FOR TEST USE

According to the 2010 CDC guidelines,[5] an IGRA may be used in place of the TST in all situations in which the TST is recommended. The CDC does not generally recommend that the IGRA be used in addition to the TST in testing and has developed certain population guidelines suggesting the use of one test type over the other.[5]

The TST is preferred over IGRAs for children younger than 5 because of the high rate of indeterminate test results in this age group and the relatively large blood sample that is needed for the IGRA.[5]

The CDC recommends the use of the IGRA for persons who have received BCG as a vaccine or for cancer therapy. The use of the IGRA in this population is expected to increase diagnostic specificity and improve the acceptance of recommended treatment for LTBI. The IGRA is also recommended in those groups in whom the return rate for having the TST read is historically low. Drug users and the homeless are 2 such groups.[5]

Testing comparing the TST with the IGRA in immunocompromised populations has not offered a clear-cut favorite between the 2 test methods when screening for latent disease. In a study performed in Zambia with 112 participants (59 infected with HIV, 37 were not infected, 16 were not HIV tested), in whom active TB was diagnosed based on sputum smear, the IGRA and TST were significantly less sensitive in persons infected with HIV. The IGRA used in the study was the QFT-GIT and in this study, the overall sensitivity for the QFT-GIT was greater than the TST (63% and 55%, respectively) in HIV-infected individuals.[6]

For those with occupational exposure to *M tuberculosis*, such as in a health care surveillance program, the CDC recommendations do not clearly support the TST or the IGRA. The recommendation is that either test may be used without preference. The advantages of the IGRA include that only 1 visit is needed to obtain results. A visit to have the TST read would necessitate a minimum of 2 visits when performing the TST. Limitations of the IGRA in this population include a greater risk of obtaining a false-positive reading.[5]

The CDC has established more rigorous criteria for determining if a TST has converted compared with that of the IGRA. The criterion defining a positive TST is an increase of ≥ 10 mm in induration within 2 years. The TST conversion is associated with an increased risk for active TB. An IGRA conversion defined as a change from negative to positive within 2 years is without any consideration to the magnitude of the change in the response and more importantly, no association between IGRA conversion and subsequent disease has been demonstrated.[5]

As noted previously, routine testing with both the TST and IGRA is not generally recommended. There are certain situations in which the results of both tests could be helpful. If an initial test is negative and the risk for infection or development of disease high or disease outcome is poor (for example in young children exposed to infectious TB), the person may benefit from a second screening test with the opposite testing method. An additional test also may be helpful in encouraging an individual to accept and adhere to treatment for LTBI if the individual is informed that both screening tests are positive. A second test also can be helpful in determining if an initial test is truly false positive or indeterminate.[5]

TESTING ADVANTAGES AND DISADVANTAGES

The limitations of the TST include low specificity. Other limitations of the TST revolve around incorrect placement of the test and poor reading results; usually due to individuals failing to return to have the test read and interpreted. Of note is that different populations have different criteria for what is considered a positive test, as outlined in Table 1. In addition, subsequent TST results can produce false-positive results because of a booster phenomenon. False-negative results also may occur in severe immunosuppressive illness, such as HIV.[5]

The IGRA, on the other hand, has reagents that are significantly more expensive and require laboratories with the appropriate equipment and adequately trained staff. The testing can be influenced by collection errors and transportation delays. In most cases, IGRAs will convert in 4 to 7 weeks after exposure, but in some cases, the conversion may take more than 3 months.[5] The TST on average takes approximately the same amount of time to become positive after exposure.

Indeterminate IGRA tests are a possibility and are more likely to occur when immune suppression leads to an inadequate T-cell reaction.[5] In a study at the International Medical Center in Tokyo, Japan, the use of the IGRA was evaluated for the diagnosis of TB on patients receiving renal dialysis (a patient population in whom immune status is known to be impaired); the indeterminate IGRA rate was 24.1%.[7] A control tube is used (for mitogen evaluation) to ensure the individual being tested has an appropriately

Table 1
Centers for Disease Control and Prevention recommendations for determining positivity of tuberculin skin test

An *induration of 5 or more millimeters*	An *induration of 10 or more millimeters*	An *induration of 15 or more millimeters*
• HIV-infected persons • A recent contact of a person with TB disease • Persons with fibrotic changes on chest radiograph consistent with prior TB • Patients with organ transplants • Persons who are immuno-suppressed for other reasons (such as persons taking the equivalent of >15 mg/d of prednisone for 1 mo or longer, or taking TNF-α antagonists)	• Recent immigrants (<5 y) from high-prevalence countries • Injection drug users • Residents and employees of high-risk congregate settings • Mycobacteriology laboratory personnel • Persons with clinical conditions that place them at high risk • Children <4 y of age • Infants, children, and ado lescents exposed to adults in high-risk categories	• Positive in any person, including persons with no known risk factors for TB

Abbreviations: HIV, human immunodeficiency virus; TB, tuberculosis; TNF-α, tumor necrosis factor alpha.

From Centers for Disease Control and Prevention. Screening for tuberculosis and tuberculosis infection in high-risk populations: recommendations of the Advisory Council for the elimination of tuberculosis. MMWR Recomm Rep 1995;44(RR-11):18–34

functioning immune status when performing the IGRA. Individuals with low control (mitogen) values will have indeterminate tests and should have an evaluation of their immune status. Another reason for indeterminate test results may be related to the handling of the specimen. The IGRA results are dependent on appropriate handling of the specimen and a timed incubation period for accuracy.[8]

A positive feature of the IGRA is that it is not affected by the antigens found in the BCG vaccine and nontuberculosis mycobacterium, and is thought to have greater specificity for *M tuberculosis.* Test results can be generally available in 24 hours in contrast to the 48 to 72 hours that are needed to finalize test results with the TST. Also, with the IGRA, the follow-up visit is not necessary.[5]

THE BURDEN OF DISEASE

As important as is picking the correct test for TB screening, so is the recognition of what populations are at greatest risk of acquiring TB. Young children are most likely to develop forms of TB that are significantly severe and deadly.[9] Pediatric tuberculosis is the term given to TB in children younger than 15. Children younger than 5 tend to be the largest group of children affected by TB in the United States. Black individuals also have a disproportionate share of TB in the United States. In the United States, the rate of TB is 6.2 higher for black individuals than white individuals.[10] Approximately 4% to 6% of all TB cases reported in the United States are found in incarcerated individuals. Homeless individuals are also another population presenting as a public health concern for TB. International travel and those immigrating from countries with high burdens of TB (eg, Latin America, Africa, Southeast Asia, India, Philippines) should be recognized as being at high risk for both latent and active disease.[1] Immigration from countries of high TB burden places this group at a greater risk of acquiring multidrug-resistant (MDR) or extensively drug-resistant disease (XDR).[1] Pregnant women are also at increased risk of acquiring TB. This risk extends into the first 6 months of the postpartum period as well.[11]

TREATMENT

The CDC has established treatment guidelines for both LTBI and active disease, suggesting a reason to test an individual for TB is in fact a reason to treat the person for either condition. Treatment guidelines for active disease are complex and must consider and rely on drug-susceptibility studies. The overall goals for the treatment of active TB are to cure the individual and to minimize the transmission of TB to others.[3] To maximize both of these goals, it is important that therapy is well supervised so the infected individual will adhere to treatment and complete the entire course of therapy. Strategies in which an adherence plan includes direct observed therapy (DOT) have been found to have higher rates of completion than those not using this strategy. Because of this fact, health departments throughout the United States employ this strategy. The responsibility for TB control and prevention in the United States rests on the public health system on the federal, state, and local agencies. The deterioration of public health programs focused on TB control in the United States is thought to have led to a resurgence of the disease during 1985 to 1992. Since 1992, funding has been increased for TB control programs, leading to a decrease in the national incidence.[10]

Currently, there are 10 drugs approved by the FDA for treating active TB. Of the approved drugs, the following medications form the backbone of core TB treatment:

- Isoniazid (INH)
- Rifampin (RIF)
- Ethambutol (EMB)
- Pyrazinamide (PZA)

The preferred treatment includes an initial phase of daily INH, RIF, PZA, and EMB for 56 doses or 8 weeks.[12] Ethambutol can be discontinued if drug-susceptibility studies prove that the TB is sensitive to the core agents INH and RIF. In the preferred treatment regimen, therapy is continued daily with INH and RIF for an additional 126 doses or 18 weeks. The 18-week continuation program is used in most patients. The following patients must remain on treatment for a 7-month continuation phase[12]:

- Patients with cavitary pulmonary TB caused by drug-susceptible organisms but who continue to have positive sputum cultures after completing 2 months of therapy.
- Patients whose initial phase of treatment did not include PZA.
- Patients who followed an alternative regimen of treatment of once-weekly INH and RIF and whose sputum culture obtained at the end of the initial phase remains positive.

Several medications are used as second-line therapies. Although not FDA approved for treatment of TB, the quinolones are commonly used to treat drug-resistant disease. In addition, because of the many drug interactions that are common to RIF, rifabutin may be used as a substitute to RIF in the treatment of TB.[12]

Several other drugs are used in the treatment of TB, and several combination agents are also available. Unfortunately, several of the agents are associated with unpleasant side effects and serious health risks, such as hepatatoxicity.[12]

Treatment completion is dependent on the total number of doses taken of each medication and not the duration of therapy. Toxicities and interruptions in therapy can necessitate treatment be restarted or substantially lengthened in duration.[12] Unfortunately, even when treatment guidelines are followed and the infected individual completes optimal treatment, the rate of reinfection disease is up to 7 times the crude incidence rate and approximately 4 times the age-adjusted incidence rate of new TB.[13] This suggests that individuals who have been successfully treated for TB are at an increased risk of developing TB again, rather than being protected from the disease.[13] Patients with cavitary disease on an initial radiograph and who have positive cultures at the end of 2 months of therapy are known to be at risk of relapse.[12]

The treatment of LTBI began in the late 1950s. At that time, a pediatrician, Edith Lincoln, began efforts at Bellevue Hospital to prevent progression of primary TB to TB meningitis among exposed children. Dr Lincoln's work and other pioneers in the field led to recommendations by the US Public Health Service and the National Tuberculosis Association to recommend chemotherapy to preventive active TB.[14]

There are currently 4 treatment regimens recommended by the CDC for LTBI. The antibiotic options include INH, rifapentine (RPT), or RIF. The standard treatment regimen for LTBI is 9 months of INH given daily. The therapy is preferred for most adults and for children ages 2 to 11 years. For patients infected with HIV and prescribed antiretroviral therapy, daily INH for 9 months also is preferred. A potential side effect of INH is peripheral neuropathy. It is relatively uncommon (<0.2% of individuals taking INH at a conventional dose) unless the individual prescribed the medication has a comorbid condition that is also associated with neuropathy (eg, diabetes, HIV, renal failure, or alcoholism). In these populations, pyridoxine (vitamin B6) supplementation is recommended. It is also recommended in patients who are pregnant.[15] The side effects of the medications commonly used to treat LTBI are listed in Box 1. INH also can be used twice weekly DOT with a minimum of 52 doses needed for treatment to be considered effective. Another effective option is a 12-dose treatment plan of INH and RPT. The medications are given weekly and administered under direct observation of medical personnel. This regimen is recommended for healthy individuals older than 12 with a greater likelihood of developing active disease. Such individuals would include persons who were recently exposed to contagious active TB who have converted their TST or IGRA testing.[15] This treatment is not recommended for persons with HIV who are on antiretroviral therapy, pregnant women, or those expecting to conceive. RIF can be used daily for 4 months as well. Treatment must be modified if the patient has had contact with an individual with drug-resistant TB disease. If the TB infection is suspected to be caused by a drug-resistant organism, it is advised that the individual be referred to a specialist in TB care for management.[15]

INH was the first antitubercular agent to be successfully used for preventive therapy. The duration of treatment for LTBI with INH has been investigated at length. The maximal beneficial effect of INH is thought to be achieved by 9 months with only minimal therapeutic gain with extended therapy. The CDC currently recommends that LTBI be treated for 9 months when using INH.[16]

INH hepatotoxicity along with the declining cost of rifampin and the drug's potent sterilization affects has led it to be used for preventive therapy as a single agent or in combination with INH. Alone or in combination therapy, the rifampin treatments are shorter than the current 9-month INH recommendation and thought to promote compliance to therapy.[16]

Box 1
Centers for Disease Control and Prevention medication side-effects profile

Possible adverse effects of isoniazid (INH)

- Asymptomatic elevation of serum liver enzyme concentrations occurs in 10%–20% of people taking INH; and liver enzyme concentrations usually return to normal even when treatment is continued. It is generally recommended that INH be withheld if a patient's transaminase level exceeds 3 times the upper limit of normal if associated with symptoms or 5 times the upper limit of normal if the patient is asymptomatic.

- Clinical hepatitis occurs in approximately 0.1% of people taking INH, and is more common when INH is combined with other hepatotoxic agents. Factors that may increase either of these rates or the severity of hepatitis include daily alcohol consumption, underlying liver disease or risks for liver disease, and the concurrent use of other medications that are metabolized in the liver. Symptomatic hepatitis is rare in patients younger than 20 years, but severe and fatal cases have been reported. Younger patients with underlying risk factors for liver disease should be monitored clinically with the same precautions as older patients.

- Peripheral neuropathy occurs in fewer than 0.2% of people taking INH at conventional doses. It is more likely in the presence of other conditions associated with neuropathy, such as diabetes, HIV, renal failure, and alcoholism. Pyridoxine (vitamin B6) supplementation is recommended only in such conditions or to prevent neuropathy in pregnant or breastfeeding women.

Possible adverse effects of rifampin (RIF) and rifapentine (RPT)

- Hepatotoxicity, evidenced by transient asymptomatic hyperbilirubinemia, may occur in 0.6% of persons taking RIF. Hepatitis is more likely when RIF is combined with INH.

- Cutaneous reactions, such as pruritis (with or without a rash), may occur in 6% of persons taking RIF. They are generally self-limited and may not be a true hypersensitivity; continued treatment may be possible.

- Rarely, rifamycins can be associated with hypersensitivity reactions, including hypotension, nephritis or thrombocytopenia, and manifested *by symptoms such as fever, headache, dizziness/lightheadedness, musculoskeletal pain, petechiae, and pruritis.*

- Gastrointestinal symptoms, such as nausea, anorexia, and abdominal pain, are rarely severe enough to discontinue treatment.

- Orange discoloration of body fluids is expected and harmless, but patients should be advised beforehand. Soft contact lenses and dentures may be permanently stained.

- RIF and RPT interact with a number of drugs, causing drug-drug interactions. They are known to reduce concentrations of methadone, warfarin, hormonal contraceptives, and phenytoin. Women using hormonal contraceptives should be advised to consider an alternative method of contraception (eg, a barrier method).

Adapted from Centers for Disease Control and Prevention. Treatment Regimens for latent TB infection (LTBI). Available at: http://www.cdc.gov/tb/topic/treatment/ltbi.htm. Accessed August 18, 2016

SUMMARY

Historical records indicate that *M tuberculosis* infection dates back to antiquity. Historical records also indicate that as hygiene and the standard of living improved, the incidence of TB declined. Unfortunately, prosperity and improved living conditions have not been afforded to all peoples. Efforts to actively treat LTBI are also not a priority in many resource-poor countries. In a resource-rich environment like the United States, a TB reduction plan that includes appropriate use of antitubercular therapy along with DOT for treatment of active TB and more rigorous efforts to identify and treat LTBI should be successful in reducing and significantly lowering the development of new TB cases. To reach TB eradication goals in the United States, all health care providers should be well versed in the diagnosis and treatment of both LTBI and active disease or be familiar with TB experts who can be used for consultation.

REFERENCES

1. Scott C, Kirking HL, Jeffreis C, et al, Centers for Disease Control and Prevention (CDC). Tuberculosis trends-United States, 2014. MMWR Morb Mortal Wkly Rep 2015;64(10):265–9.
2. Ioachimescu OC, Tomford JW. Tuberculosis. In: Carey WD, editor. Current clinical medicine. 2nd edition. Philadelphia: Saunders; 2009. p. 758–64.
3. Centers for Disease Control and Prevention. Screening for tuberculosis and tuberculosis infection in high-risk populations: recommendations of the advisory council for the elimination of tuberculosis. MMWR Recomm Rep 1995;44(RR-11): 18–34.
4. Testing for TB Infection. Centers for Disease Control and Prevention Web site. Available at: http://www.cdc.gov/tb/topic/testing/tbtesttypes.htm. Accessed August 17, 2016.
5. Centers for Disease Control and Prevention. Updated guidelines for using interferon gamma release assays to detect *Mycobacterium tuberculosis* infection - United States, 2010. MMWR Recomm Rep 2010;59(RR-5):1–25.
6. Raby E, Moyo M, Devendra A, et al. The effects of HIV on the sensitivity of a whole blood IFN-γ release assay in Zambian adults with active tuberculosis. PLoS One 2008;3(6):e2489.
7. Inoue I, Nakamura T, Katsuma A, et al. The value of Quantiferon TB-Gold in the diagnosis of tuberculosis among dialysis patients. Nephrol Dial Transplant 2009;24(7): 2252–7.
8. Pai M, Menzies D. Interferon-gamma release assays for diagnosis of latent tuberculosis infection. In: von Reyn CF, editor. UpToDate. Waltham (MA): UpToDate; 2016. p. 1–8.
9. Tuberculosis in Children in the United States. Centers for Disease Control and Prevention Web site. 2014. Available at: http://www.cdc.gov/tb/topic/populations/tbinchildren/default.htm. Accessed October 3, 2016.
10. Centers for Disease Control and Prevention. Controlling tuberculosis in the United States: recommendations from the American Thoracic Society, CDC, and the Infectious Diseases Society of America. MMWR Recomm Rep 2005;54(RR-12): 1–82.
11. Zenner D, Kruijshaar ME, Andrews N, et al. Risk of tuberculosis in pregnancy. Am J Respir Crit Care Med 2012;185(7):779–84.
12. American Thoracic Society, CDC, Infectious Diseases Society of America. Treatment of tuberculosis. MMWR Recomm Rep 2003;52(RR-11):1–77.
13. Verver S, Warren RM, Beyers N, et al. Rate of reinfection tuberculosis after treatment is higher than rate of new infection. Am J Respir Crit Care Med 2005;171(12): 1430–5.
14. Donald P. Edith Lincoln, an American pioneer in childhood tuberculosis. Pediatr Infect Dis J 2013;32(3):241–5.
15. Treatment Regimens for latent TB infection (LTBI). Centers for Disease Control and Prevention Web site. 2016. Available at: http://www.cdc.gov/tb/topic/treatment/ltbi.htm. Accessed August 18, 2016.
16. Targeted tuberculin testing and treatment of latent tuberculosis infection. American Thoracic Society. MMWR Recomm Rep 2000;49(RR06):1–51.

Infectious Diarrhea

Christopher Roman, PA-C, MA, MMS[a],*, Tia Solh, PA-C, MT(ASCP), MPAS[b],
Mary Broadhurst, PA-C, MPAS[c]

KEYWORDS

- Diarrhea • Dehydration • Norovirus • Campylobacter • Salmonella • Shigella
- Shiga toxin-producing E coli • Parasites

KEY POINTS

- Patients complaining of diarrheal illness without bloody and/or mucoid stools may use antimotility agents, but patients with bloody and/or mucoid stools should refrain from using these medications.
- Significant dehydration is the most common complication of diarrhea. Rehydration is the cornerstone of management for patients with diarrhea, regardless of any other ongoing therapies (eg, antimicrobials).
- Diagnostic tests are not needed for most cases of diarrhea, as it tends to be a benign, self-limited problem. Diagnostics are appropriate in some situations, such as an immunocompromised host, prolonged course of illness, or inflammatory diarrhea.

INTRODUCTION

Diarrhea, an increase in stool frequency and/or liquidity, causes 1.5 million deaths per year across the globe,[1] including 750,000 children younger than 5 years.[2] Much of this burden of disease affects poor nations and is caused by improper hygiene, poor sanitation, or unsafe water supplies. These risk factors are generally minimized in countries with greater resources, and diarrheal illnesses are rarely fatal in such locations. In the United States, there are more than 200 million cases of diarrheal illness annually.[3] Although mortality is much lower in more affluent countries, it remains an important cause of lost productivity and the complaint in more than 8 million clinic visits annually.[4]

There are many pathogens that can cause diarrhea, and many (but not all) of these organisms are reviewed in this article. Broadly, these may be considered as viral (*Norovirus* is discussed later), bacterial (*Campylobacter*, *Salmonella*, *Shigella*, and Shiga toxin–producing *Escherichia coli*), or parasitic (*Cryptosporidium* and *Giardia*)

Disclosure Statement: The authors have nothing to disclose.
[a] Department of Physician Assistant Studies, Butler University, 4600 Sunset Avenue, Indianapolis, IN 46208, USA; [b] Department of Physician Assistant Studies, Mercer University, 3001 Mercer University Drive, Atlanta, GA 30341, USA; [c] Department of Infectious Diseases, Saint Vincent Hospital, 2001 West 86th Street, Indianapolis, IN 46260, USA
* Corresponding author.
E-mail address: croman@butler.edu

Physician Assist Clin 2 (2017) 229–245
http://dx.doi.org/10.1016/j.cpha.2016.12.006
2405-7991/17/© 2016 Elsevier Inc. All rights reserved.

physicianassistant.theclinics.com

infections. Careful history taking and physical examination are key to identifying the likely cause and severity of a case of infectious diarrhea and the selection of appropriate diagnostic and therapeutic interventions. Several important causes of diarrheal illness, including *Clostridium difficile* and *Rotavirus*, are not included in this review as they merit a more expansive discussion than can be included here.

Inflammation

Inflammatory diarrhea, also known as dysentery, results from pathogens that classically affect the distal ileum and colon, where they invade the epithelium or release toxins. This invasion results in febrile diarrheal illness with small stool volume, tenesmus, and stools with blood, leukocytes, and/or mucus. Noninflammatory diarrhea is caused by organisms that generally affect the small intestine and cause larger-volume stools without fever, tenesmus, fecal blood, leukocytes, or mucus.[5]

Severity of Dehydration

Traditionally, the degree of dehydration has been determined by the presence and degree of symptoms and the magnitude (in percent) of volume deficit. Mild dehydration (<3%–5%) is generally asymptomatic; moderate (5%–10%) dehydration will have some symptoms, such as dry mucous membranes and increased thirst; severe (>10%) dehydration will have numerous signs and symptoms, including electrolyte abnormalities and hemodynamic instability. Recent guidelines have combined mild and moderate dehydration to allow for some variability in the presence of symptoms in patients with less than 10% volume deficit.[6]

General Approach to Evaluation

A detailed history and physical examination are indispensable to the evaluation of patients with diarrhea. Stool testing is not needed for most cases of infectious diarrhea, as most are self-limited. However, in cases of inflammatory or protracted diarrhea, diagnostics are appropriate. General testing modalities are mainly geared toward identifying inflammation (fecal leukocytes, fecal lactoferrin, or fecal occult blood) or fecal ova and parasites.[3] Testing for inflammation is appropriate for individuals with one or more the following[3]:

- Bloody stools
- Fever
- Tenesmus
- Recent antibiotics
- Day care center attendance
- Hospitalization
- Moderate to severe dehydration

More specialized testing for specific organisms and/or toxins may be appropriate in some cases; these are discussed in the relevant sections of this article. Stool cultures are invaluable for identification of bacterial pathogens and are the cornerstone of diagnostics for these organisms. Many laboratories are also using polymerase chain reaction (PCR) testing, as this can yield faster confirmation and higher sensitivity/specificity than culture. For patients hospitalized longer than 3 days who are not elderly or immunocompromised, stool cultures are very unlikely to yield an enteric pathogen other than *Clostridium difficile*.[3] Testing for parasitic infections, such as *Giardia* and *Cryptosporidium*, are appropriate for episodes of diarrhea lasting longer than 7 days or with risk factors for these infections.[3] To reduce the spread of disease, food handlers and health care workers should demonstrate 2 consecutive negative stool samples and resolution of symptoms for at least 48 hours before returning to work.[3]

General Approach to Treatment

The mainstay of therapy for all diarrheal illnesses is supportive care, consisting of fluid and electrolyte replacement to prevent dehydration.[3,6,7] The Centers for Disease Control and Prevention recommends 60 to 120 mL of oral rehydration solution (ORS) per episode of vomiting or diarrhea for children less than 10 kg and 120 to 140 mL of ORS per episode for children weighing more than 10 kg.[6] Commercial oral rehydration solutions may be used; but fluids such as sports drinks and fruit juice should be avoided, though juices may be diluted 50/50 with water and used as ORS.[8] In children with more than 10% body weight loss due to dehydration, intravenous (IV) fluids are recommended, beginning with a 20-mL/kg bolus.[6]

Indications for hospitalization of individuals with acute diarrheal illness include[7] the following:

- Shock or toxicity
- Neurologic involvement
- Severe dehydration
- Moderate dehydration with inability to tolerate oral fluids or failure of oral rehydration therapy
- Malnutrition or immunodeficiency
- Infants younger than 3 months

Antimotility agents, such as loperamide, should not be used for patients with signs of inflammatory diarrhea (eg, fever, bloody stools)[3] but can generally be used for noninflammatory episodes of diarrhea. The decision to implement antimicrobial therapy should only occur with either a firm diagnosis or high suspicion for a particular pathogen (ie, traveler's diarrhea, shigellosis, and campylobacter infection).[3] Such therapeutic options are mentioned in the relevant section for each pathogen. Probiotics also have a modest role in decreasing incidence and severity of infectious diarrheal illnesses. It is important to counsel patients on the importance of prevention for diarrheal illnesses, such as handwashing, avoiding undercooked meat/seafood and unpasteurized dairy products, and vaccinating against typhoid when traveling to endemic areas.[3]

VIRAL CAUSES OF DIARRHEA

Viral gastroenteritis is usually a self-limiting illness of short duration characterized by abrupt-onset vomiting and diarrhea. Four groups of viruses have been identified as important causes of gastroenteritis: rotaviruses, noroviruses, astroviruses, and the enteric adenoviruses. These groups share several features, including fecal-oral spread, brief incubation periods, and epidemic or sporadic outbreaks.

This section focuses on the human noroviruses, which belong to the family of caliciviruses. The first recognized norovirus outbreak occurred at a school in Norwalk, Ohio in 1968; thus, the virus used to be called the Norwalk agent. Noroviruses are nonenveloped, single-stranded RNA viruses composed of 6 genogroups, with most human infections resulting from genogroups GI and GII.[9,10]

Epidemiology, Risk Factors, and Transmission

Norovirus is the leading cause of epidemic outbreaks of acute gastroenteritis across all age groups, both in the United States and worldwide.[11] Globally, norovirus is the second most common cause of diarrheal death in children younger than 5 years and is responsible for 200,000 deaths in developing countries each year. In the United States, the elderly are at greatest risk of death due to norovirus, but the highest number of norovirus-related medical visits are composed of children less than 5 years of age.[11,12] In the United States, norovirus causes about 20 million illnesses, 400,000 visits to the emergency department, 60,000 hospitalizations, and up to 800 deaths annually.[11]

Norovirus infections occur year-round but peak in the winter months. As few as 18 virus particles can cause infection; the virus is able to spread easily in areas of confinement, such as cruise ships, long-term care facilities, schools, and day care centers.[13] The virus spreads through several transmission routes, including directly from person to person (fecal-oral and vomitus-oral) and indirectly through fecally contaminated fomites, food, or water. Most cases are due to direct transmission, and vomiting is strongly associated with transmission because of the spread of aerosolized viral particles during emesis.[9,10] Infected persons handling ready-to-eat foods, such as leafy vegetables, fruits, and shellfish, are the most common cause of foodborne norovirus outbreaks.[9] Noroviruses are notoriously resilient and have caused infection after remaining in groundwater for more than 60 days. Similar studies have shown that norovirus is potentially infectious on frozen foods for up to 6 months and on fomites for up to 14 days.[9] Further contributing to transmission, up to 30% of patients shed the virus before developing symptoms; shedding can last several weeks, long after symptoms have resolved.[7]

Clinical Manifestations

After an incubation period of 12 to 48 hours, illness in the immunocompetent individual is usually abrupt in onset and self-limiting, lasting 2 to 3 days. Clinical manifestations include nausea, vomiting, cramping, malaise, myalgias, and diarrhea. Most patients develop both vomiting and diarrhea, though either manifestation can present alone. Fever can occur in up to half of patients. Common sequelae include hypovolemia and electrolyte imbalances, which can be further complicated by hypokalemia and renal insufficiency.[10] Stools are usually watery and nonbloody.

Severe outcomes and longer durations of illness are more likely in the elderly, hospitalized patients with multiple comorbidities, and the immunocompromised.[10] Norovirus can cause prolonged shedding and persistent infection in immunocompromised patients, lasting from weeks to years, and resulting in debilitating disease and death. Chronic norovirus infection has been reported in patients after organ transplantation as well as in patients with human immunodeficiency virus (HIV) and cancer.[14] Noroviruses in chronically infected immunocompromised patients have been shown to change their antigenic profile over time by altering their amino acids on the outer surface of their capsids.[14]

Diagnostic Evaluation

Laboratory testing for patients with vomiting and diarrhea suspected to be caused by viral illness is typically not performed, as the diagnosis is usually clinical. In addition, the presence of fecal leukocytes and leukocytosis is uncommon in patients with norovirus infection.[7] However, confirmation of norovirus may be needed for epidemiologic purposes or for patients who are immunocompromised. The current gold standard for confirmation is reverse transcriptase PCR (RT-PCR).[10,12] However, clinical laboratories may use less effective methods like enzyme immunoassays (EIA) or electron microscopy, as RT-PCR is not widely available.[10]

Management

As with all diarrheal illnesses, ensuring adequate hydration is the cornerstone of therapy for norovirus infections. Management of norovirus outbreaks in a health care setting includes proper hand hygiene, contact precautions, and enhanced environmental cleaning and disinfection procedures.[9] Licensed vaccines for noroviruses do not yet exist, but the development and evaluation of recombinant viruslike particle vaccines is underway.

BACTERIAL CAUSES OF DIARRHEA

All of the bacterial pathogens discussed here are nationally notifiable conditions that should be reported when identified in clinical practice.[15]

CAMPYLOBACTER
Epidemiology, Risk Factors, and Transmission

Campylobacter species are gram-negative rods with a gull-wing appearance on gram stain. These pathogens are found in virtually all climates globally, reside in most bodies of water, and heavily colonize agricultural animals (especially birds). There are more than 20 different *Campylobacter* species; of these, *Campylobacter jejuni* is the most common offender (66%).[16] After *Salmonella*, it is the most common bacterial cause of diarrhea in the United States with an incidence of 16 per 100,000 person-years,[17] although some studies have suggested the numbers to be much greater.[18]

Infection typically occurs following ingestion of contaminated food or liquid, with the most common risk factors being consumption of poultry (especially chicken), raw milk, contaminated water, or contact with animals.[16] Gastric acidity is protective against campylobacter infection, and usage of proton-pump inhibitors is associated with a 10-fold increased risk of infection.[19]

Clinical Manifestations

After an incubation period of 3 days, 30% of campylobacter infections manifests as a febrile prodrome with headache, dizziness, or myalgias without abdominal symptoms.[20] This prodrome is subsequently followed by diarrhea (<30% with blood) and continuous, often severe abdominal pain, which may manifest with peritoneal signs.[20] Because up to 30% of children infected with *Campylobacter* may not have diarrhea, this abdominal pain may be confused with appendicitis or other causes of abdominal pain.[20] Most patients with *Campylobacter* experience fairly mild, self-limited disease. Diarrhea persists for a mean of 7 days,[21] with shedding of bacteria in the stools for several weeks.

Campylobacter is the most common cause of Guillain-Barré syndrome (GBS), an immune-mediated peripheral polyneuropathy that manifests as ascending weakness and paralysis.[22] It has been estimated that *Campylobacter* causes 30% to 40% of cases of GBS[23]; this can occur even with asymptomatic infections.[24] Reactive arthritis (formerly known as Reiter syndrome) is another recognized complication of campylobacter infections. This syndrome of arthritis, uveitis, and urethritis manifests in 1% to 5% of patients infected with *Campylobacter*.[25]

Diagnostic Evaluation

As mentioned earlier, stool culture and/or PCR testing is essential in diagnosing bacterial diarrheal infections, including *Campylobacter*.

Treatment

Antimicrobial therapy directed at campylobacter infection can shorten the duration of symptoms by 1 to 2 days.[3] In addition to rehydration, therapeutic options include azithromycin (500 mg orally daily) or, if susceptible to fluoroquinolones (resistance is a growing problem), ciprofloxacin (500 mg orally twice daily) or levofloxacin (500 mg orally daily).[26–28] Treatment generally lasts 3 days or until clinical improvement occurs, and 7 to 14 days of therapy is common for immunocompromised patients.

SALMONELLA

Salmonella is a gram-negative facultative anaerobe. Salmonella infections can be broadly divided as typhoidal (*S typhi* or *paratyphi*) infections that cause typhoid fever or nontyphoidal infections with other serotypes that generally cause gastrointestinal illness. For ease of reading, these are considered separately here.

Nontyphoidal Salmonella

Epidemiology, risk factors, and transmission

Nontyphoidal *Salmonella* is the most commonly identified cause of foodborne gastroenteritis in the United States[17] and causes approximately 100 million infections globally each year with 155,000 deaths.[29] Internationally, salmonella infections are transmitted in areas of poor sanitation and hygiene; shedding of the pathogen is common during convalescence and in asymptomatic infections.[30]

Salmonella outbreaks have been reported from alfalfa,[31] eggs,[32] ice cream,[33] poultry,[34] contaminated water,[35] and others.

Clinical manifestations

Nontyphoidal salmonella infections typically cause a self-limited gastrointestinal illness with fever, nausea, abdominal pain, and diarrhea that may or may not be bloody. These symptoms arise after an incubation period of approximately 24 hours and last a mean of 7 days.[32] About 3% of nontyphoidal salmonella infections become invasive with bacteremia, endocarditis, osteomyelitis, or others.[35] Although salmonella osteomyelitis is rare in the general population, it is the most common cause of osteomyelitis in children with sickle cell disease.[36]

Diagnostic evaluation

As mentioned earlier, stool culture and/or PCR testing is essential in diagnosing bacterial diarrheal infections, including nontyphoidal *Salmonella*. Urinalysis and urine culture are frequently part of the workup for febrile patients; urine cultures revealing *Salmonella* should prompt evaluation for bacteremia and an endovascular infection.[37]

Management

Antibiotic therapy may be initiated for those with severe disease (>9 stools daily, persistent fever, inpatient therapy), risk of invasive disease (eg, immunosuppression, prosthetic cardiac valve), or typhoid fever. Therapeutic options for *Salmonella* (both typhoidal and nontyphoidal) include fluoroquinolones (ciprofloxacin 500 mg twice daily for 7 days or levofloxacin 500 mg daily for 7 days) or ceftriaxone 1 to 2 g IV daily for 7 days.[3]

Typhoidal Salmonella

Epidemiology, risk factors, and transmission

Typhoid fever (also known as enteric fever) is a prominent infection globally, causing more than 20 million cases and 200,000 deaths each year.[38] In the United States, there are approximately 300 cases per year, mostly in returning travelers from endemic areas where contaminated food/beverages and sanitation issues cause most cases of transmission.[38,39]

Clinical manifestations

Following a 1- to 2-week incubation after ingestion, typhoid fever classically manifests with fever, abdominal pain, headache, hepatosplenomegaly, and a rose spot rash.[40] Constipation is more common in adults, whereas diarrhea predominates in children and patients with HIV. Severe disease can result in intestinal hemorrhage or perforation, meningitis, or myocarditis.[40]

Diagnostic evaluation

Blood cultures are the most common diagnostic approach, though bone marrow culture is more sensitive.[40] Stool cultures are only positive in 30% of patients.[40] PCR testing for typhoidal Salmonella is being developed but is not yet widely available.[41]

Management

Antibiotic approaches to treating typhoidal *Salmonella* are discussed earlier with non-typhoidal organisms. Vaccination is recommended against typhoid fever for individuals preparing to travel to endemic areas, virtually all of the developing countries in the world where problems with sanitation and public health remain.[3,42]

SHIGELLA

Epidemiology, Risk Factors, and Transmission

After *Salmonella* and *Campylobacter*, *Shigella* is the most common foodborne diarrheal illness in the United States.[17] An inoculum of as few as 10 of these gram-negative rods can be sufficient to cause disease[43,44]; this can occur through ingestion of contaminated foods, poor sanitation, or through contact with affected individuals (fecal-oral spread).[45] Spread through contact has important epidemiologic implications: children younger than 9 years are approximately 500% more likely to contract *Shigella* than older individuals,[17] presumably because of their close quarters in day care centers and schools. An additional mode of transmission is sexual contact among men who have sex with men, particularly those who are HIV positive.[46]

Clinical Manifestations

The mean incubation period for shigellosis is 3 days. Whereas the diarrheal illnesses caused by *Campylobacter* and *Salmonella* display variable amounts of inflammation, *Shigella* is more likely to manifest with the classic signs of an inflammatory diarrhea: fever, abdominal pain, tenesmus, and mucoid (33%–86%) and/or bloody (25%–55%) stools.[3,47–50] Because this pathogen initially affects the small intestine before transitioning to the colon, stools are watery and voluminous early in the infection before becoming small-volume but frequent.

One of the most common complications of shigellosis (up to 40% of pediatric cases) is the development of neurologic changes that can include encephalopathy and self-limited seizures.[51,52] Intestinal complications can include proctitis, obstruction, toxic megacolon, or perforation. Relatively rare findings include bacteremia,[53] reactive arthritis,[54] and hemolytic-uremic syndrome (HUS, discussed separately later).

Diagnostic Evaluation

As mentioned earlier, stool culture and/or PCR testing is essential in diagnosing bacterial diarrheal infections, including *Shigella*.

Management

Antibiotic therapy can reduce the duration of illness and bacterial shedding and is recommended for all patients with confirmed shigellosis. Fluoroquinolones (ciprofloxacin 500 mg twice daily or levofloxacin 500 mg daily for 3 days) have been the mainstay of therapy.[3] In pediatric cases, or individuals that cannot take fluoroquinolones, other options include azithromycin, ceftriaxone, or trimethoprim-sulfamethoxazole (if susceptibility is confirmed).[3] Resistance rates against many of these antibiotics are increasing, particularly in Africa and Asia, so antibiotic susceptibility testing is essential to guiding therapy.[55]

SHIGA TOXIN AND HEMOLYTIC UREMIC SYNDROME

Shigella organisms elaborate several toxins, but Shiga-toxin (Stx) is the most potent. Stx-producing Escherichia coli (STEC) organisms elaborate similar toxins (see later discussion). Although Stx increases intestinal secretion and sometimes causes intestinal hemorrhage, it is not essential for these pathogens to cause diarrhea. However, they are the primary cause of postdiarrheal development of the HUS.[56]

This thrombotic microangiopathy presents similarly to thrombotic thrombocytopenic purpura. It is associated with hemolytic anemia, thrombocytopenia, and organ dysfunction that most commonly presents as renal insufficiency.[57] Extrarenal manifestations of HUS are frequently reported, with neurologic manifestations being the most serious.[58] HUS is most common in children younger than 5 years, and approximately 90% of cases are caused by STEC.[59] Shigella infection can also cause HUS, as can Streptococcus pneumoniae and others. Treatment of HUS focuses on addressing the hematologic and renal manifestations: transfusions of red blood cells and/or platelets, adjusting medications for renal impairment, and possibly hemodialysis.

SHIGA TOXIN–PRODUCING ESCHERICHIA COLI
Epidemiology, Risk Factors, Transmission, and Clinical Manifestations

Although notorious as a cause of HUS, STEC is also a frequent cause of dysentery, accounting for 15% to 36% of episodes of bloody diarrhea.[59] Foodborne outbreaks have arisen after distribution of contaminated fenugreek sprouts,[60] spinach,[61] water,[62] and most famously, beef.[63,64] These pathogenic strains of E coli are typed based on 2 antigens: O and H. The most important and best studied of these is E coli O157:H7, which was identified in the famous 1993 outbreak from contaminated beef at Jack in the Box restaurants.[64] Numerous other subtypes exist that may cause dysentery and HUS.

Diagnostic Evaluation

Testing for STEC (specifically E coli O157:H7) is appropriate for all cases of acute bloody diarrhea and/or HUS.[3] Because STEC is difficult to culture, agglutination or PCR testing for Stx-1 and Stx-2 is the usual method to detect STEC.[3]

Management

Once identified, the therapeutic approach for STEC depends on the bacterial type. Although trimethoprim-sulfamethoxazole and fluoroquinolones are effective against pathogenic E coli, the role of antibiotics in STEC is controversial.[3] Current guidelines discourage the use of antimotility agents and antimicrobial therapy in STEC infections.[3] This recommendation is based on numerous demonstrations that several antibiotics (including quinolones and trimethoprim-sulfamethoxazole) increase Stx production in these pathogens, which elevates the risk of HUS.[3,65,66] Treatment, therefore, centers on hydration and careful observation for sequelae, such as HUS.[65]

PARASITIC CAUSES OF DIARRHEA

Both of the parasites discussed here are nationally notifiable conditions that should be reported when identified in clinical practice.[15]

GIARDIA
Epidemiology, Risk Factors, and Transmission

Giardia duodenalis, also known as *G intestinalis* or *G lamblia*, is a flagellated protozoan parasite. Several other species of *Giardia* do exist; however, only *G duodenalis* is known to infect human beings and trigger the diarrheal illness known as giardiasis.[67]

Giardiasis occurs across the globe, with highest rates of infection in the developing nations.[67] Although most cases are sporadic,[67] outbreaks do occur and are increasingly being documented worldwide.[68] In the United States, the incidence of giardiasis has decreased during recent years with only 15,223 new cases reported in 2012.[69] Rates of infection remain highest in the northern states, and cases of giardiasis peak in the summer months of July and August.[69] There is a bimodal age distribution affecting those aged 1 to 9 years and 45 to 49 years the greatest.[69]

G duodenalis is spread by the fecal-oral route mainly through the ingestion of contaminated water and food.[70–75] Although both human beings and animals serve as hosts for *Giardia*,[67] limited data exist regarding the significance of zoonotic transmission.[67,76,77] Any activity in which exposure to contaminated water is possible may increase the risk of acquiring giardiasis, such as consuming water from shallow wells,[78] drinking tap water, or swimming in a contaminated body of water.[79] Increased risk of acquiring giardiasis is also associated with poor sanitation, younger age, foreign travel, camping, and contact with day care attendees.[78,80]

Clinical Manifestations

Giardiasis may be asymptomatic or cause a diarrheal illness that may be acute or, rarely, chronic. In symptomatic disease, there is an incubation period of 1 to 2 weeks.[81] Symptoms most commonly experienced include diarrhea, malaise, steatorrhea, flatulence, abdominal cramps and bloating, nausea, weight loss, and vomiting.[81] Symptoms typically resolve in 2 to 4 weeks; but chronic disease may occur, particularly in patients with HIV, chronic steroid use, or other immunodeficiency.[82,83] Complications of giardiasis include malabsorption of fat, vitamins, and protein[81,84]; growth retardation and poor cognitive function in children[85,86]; and a transient lactose intolerance.[81,87]

Diagnostic Evaluation

Traditionally, giardiasis was diagnosed by stool examination for ova and parasites.[88] Currently, antigen detection assays and nucleic acid amplification tests are the preferred method for diagnosis because of their high sensitivity and rapid results.[88,89]

Management

First-line drug options for the treatment of symptomatic giardiasis include metronidazole, tinidazole, or nitazoxanide.[90,91] Second-line options include albendazole, mebendazole, or paromomycin.[90,91] Paromomycin is the current drug of choice during pregnancy.[90] Prevention of parasitic infectious diarrhea is advised by practicing good hand hygiene and sanitation as well as avoidance of contaminated or untreated drinking water.

CRYPTOSPORIDIUM
Epidemiology, Risk Factors, and Transmission

Cryptosporidiosis is the gastrointestinal (and in some cases respiratory and biliary tract) illness caused by the intracellular protozoan parasite of the genus *Cryptosporidium*. Cryptosporidiosis has been documented on every human-occupied continent in the world,[92] with historically higher prevalence in the developing countries.[93] In the United States, incidence of the disease dramatically increased during 2005 to 2012 compared with prior years,[94] with a peak incidence of 11,657 cases in 2007.[95] Whether this increase is due to an actual increase in disease transmission or better disease recognition, diagnostic testing, and reporting is yet to be determined.[94] Infection rates are highest in the Midwest and peak during August.[94] Those aged between 1 and 4 years are impacted the most by this disease, followed by those aged 5 to 9 years and 25 to 29 years, respectively.[94]

Cryptosporidium is transmitted primarily via the fecal-oral route through contaminated water[96–98] and food.[99] Increased risk of acquiring *Cryptosporidium* is associated with exposure to children aged 2 to 11 years with diarrhea, international travel, contact with farm animals (particularly cattle), swimming in freshwater or pools,[100] and ingesting untreated drinking water.[101]

Cryptosporidiosis remains the number one cause of recreational waterborne outbreaks of diarrheal illness in the United States.[73] Person-to-person and animal-to-person transmission has also been documented.[102]

Clinical Manifestations

Cryptosporidiosis has an average incubation period of 1 week[92]; infection may be asymptomatic, acute, chronic, or fulminant depending on the host. In the immunocompetent host, patients usually present with an acute, self-limited, nonbloody, watery diarrheal illness. Other symptoms include abdominal pain, nausea, vomiting, fever, and myalgias.[96] Spontaneous resolution without therapy occurs in 5 to 10 days.[92] Those who are immunocompromised (eg, HIV/AIDS) are at an increased risk for chronic or fulminant disease. In addition to the aforementioned symptoms, they may also experience life-threatening wasting and malabsorption.[103] Extraintestinal manifestations, such as biliary tract involvement[104] and respiratory involvement,[105] have also been documented in patients with HIV/AIDS.

Diagnostic Evaluation

The preferred methods of diagnosis include *Cryptosporidium*-specific EIA, direct fluorescent antibody (DFA), and PCR stool specimen testing because of their high specificity and sensitivity.[89,106,107] Cryptosporidiosis can still be diagnosed with traditional microscopy; however, at least 3 stool specimens must be examined and the practitioner must specifically request a modified acid-fast stain for cryptosporidium detection.

Management

In the immunocompetent host, treatment is not mandatory. If symptoms are persistent or severe, the first-line drug of choice is nitazoxanide.[90] Other agents, such as paromomycin and azithromycin, have not yet proven to be effective.[108] In immunocompromised hosts, supportive care and treatment of the primary disorder (HIV, leukemia, lymphoma, T-cell deficiency) is essential. A trial of antiparasitic medications may be attempted; however, studies have not shown efficacy in the immunocompromised population.[109]

Table 1
Presentation, diagnosis, and treatment of common diarrheal illnesses

Pathogen	Mean Incubation Period (d)	Bloody Stools	Complications	Diagnostics	First-Line Treatment
Norovirus	1	No	Dehydration	PCR	Supportive care
Campylobacter	3	Yes	Guillain-Barré	Stool culture	Azithromycin 500 mg daily
Salmonella (nontyphoid)	1	Yes	Bacteremia Endocarditis Osteomyelitis	Stool culture	Ciprofloxacin 500 mg bid Levofloxacin 500 mg daily Ceftriaxone 1–2 g daily
Salmonella (typhoid)	7–14	Uncommon	Bacteremia Intestinal hemorrhage Meningitis Myocarditis	Blood culture Bone marrow culture	Ciprofloxacin 500 mg bid Levofloxacin 500 mg daily Ceftriaxone 1–2 g daily
Shigella	3	Yes	Encephalopathy Seizures Bacteremia HUS	Stool culture	Ciprofloxacin 500 mg bid Levofloxacin 500 mg daily
Shiga toxin–producing *E coli*	3	Yes	HUS	Shiga-toxin EIA Serotyping	Supportive care (antimicrobials increase risk of HUS)
Giardia	7–14	No	Malabsorption	Giardia Antigen Nucleic acid amplification test	Metronidazole 500 mg tid
Cryptosporidium	7	No	Biliary or respiratory disease (immunocompromised) Malabsorption	EIA DFA PCR	Immunocompetent: supportive care Immunosuppressed: nitazoxanide 500 mg bid

SUMMARY

Diarrhea is a common ailment. Although infections are frequent causes of diarrheal illness, most cases are caused by viruses and are relatively benign and self-limited. Episodes of diarrhea associated with foodborne outbreaks or with unusual features, such as dysentery (bloody/mucoid stools), fever, or a prolonged course of disease, should prompt investigation for bacterial and/or parasitic pathogens. Rehydration is the cornerstone of therapy for patients with diarrheal illness, and oral rehydration is sufficient for most patients. Antimicrobial therapy is appropriate for select cases/pathogens, but diagnostic testing is essential to ensure appropriate diagnosis and treatment (Table 1).

REFERENCES

1. World Health Organization. Global Health Observatory data repository. Available at: http://apps.who.int/gho/data/node.main.CODWORLD?lang=en. Accessed June 18, 2016.
2. Liu L, Johnson HL, Sousens S, et al. Global, regional, and national causes of child mortality: an updated systemic analysis for 2010 with time trends since 2000. Lancet 2012;379(9832):2151–61.
3. Guerrant RL, Van Gilder T, Steiner TS, et al. Practice guidelines for the management of infectious diarrhea. Clin Infect Dis 2001;32(3):331–51.
4. Garthright WE, Archer DL, Kvenberg JE. Estimates of incidence and costs of intestinal infectious diseases in the United States. Public Health Rep 1988;103(2):107–15.
5. Navaneethan U, Giannella RA. Mechanisms of infectious diarrhea. Nat Clin Pract Gastroenterol Hepatol 2008;5(11):637–47.
6. King CK, Glass R, Bresce JS, et al. Managing acute gastroenteritis among children. MMWR Recomm Rep 2003;52(RR-16):1–16.
7. Getto L, Zeserson E, Breyer M. Vomiting, diarrhea, constipation, and gastroenteritis. Emerg Med Clin North Am 2011;29(2):211–37.
8. Freedman SB, Willan AR, Boutis K, et al. Effect of dilute apple juice and preferred fluids vs electrolyte maintenance solution on treatment failure among children with mild gastroenteritis: a randomized clinical trial. JAMA 2016;315(18):1966–74.
9. Barclay L, Park GW, Vega E, et al. Infection control for norovirus. Clin Microbiol Infect 2014;20:731–40.
10. MacCannell T, Umscheid C, Agarwal R, et al. Guideline for the prevention and control of norovirus gastroenteritis outbreaks in healthcare settings. Infect Control Hosp Epidemiol 2011;32(10):939–69.
11. Hall AJ, Lopman BA, Payne DC, et al. Norovirus disease in the United States. Emerg Infect Dis 2013;19:1198–205.
12. Lopman B, Steele D, Kirkwood C, et al. The vast and varied global burden of norovirus: prospects for prevention and control. PLoS Med 2016;13(4):e1001999. MEDLINE Complete, Ipswich, MA. Available at: http://dx.doi.org/10.1371/journal.pmed.1001999. Accessed June 15, 2016.
13. Debbink K, Lindesmith LC, Baric RS. The state of norovirus vaccines. Clin Infect Dis 2014;58(12):1746–52.
14. Green KY. Norovirus Infection in immunocompromised hosts. Clin Microbiol Infect 2014;20:717–23.

15. Centers for Disease Control and Prevention. 2016 Nationally notifiable conditions. Available at: https://wwwn.cdc.gov/nndss/conditions/notifiable/2016/. Accessed June 14, 2016.

16. Taylor EV, Herman KM, Ailes EC, et al. Common source outbreaks of Campylobacter infection in the USA, 1997-2008. Epidemiol Infect 2013;141(5):987–99.

17. Centers for Disease Control and Prevention. Incidence and trends of infection with pathogens transmitted commonly through food—foodborne diseases and active surveillance network, 10 U.S. sites, 1996-2012. MMWR Morb Mortal Wkly Rep 2013;62(15):283–7.

18. Blaser MJ. Epidemiologic and clinical features of Campylobacter jejuni infections. J Infect Dis 1997;176(Suppl 2):S103–5.

19. Neal KR, Scott HM, Slack RC, et al. Omeprazole as a risk factor for Campylobacter gastroenteritis: case-control study. BMJ 1996;312(7028):414–5.

20. Blaser MJ, Engberg J. Clinical aspects of Camplylobacter jejuni and Campylobacter coli infections. In: Nachamkin I, Szymanski CM, Blaser MJ, editors. Campylobacter. 3rd edition. Washington, DC: ASM Press; 2008. p. 99–122. Chapter 6.

21. Nelson JM, Smith KE, Vugia DJ, et al. Prolonged diarrhea due to ciprofloxacin-resistant Campylobacter infection. J Infect Dis 2004;190(6):1150–7.

22. Jacobs BC, van Belkum A, Endtz HP. Guillain-Barré syndrome and campylobacter infection. In: Nachamkin I, Szymanski CM, Blaser MJ, editors. Campylobacter. 3rd edition. Washington, DC: ASM Press; 2008. p. 245–62. Chapter 13.

23. Nachamkin I, Allos BM, Ho T. Campylobacter species and Guillain-Barré syndrome. Clin Microbiol Rev 1998;11(3):555.

24. Kalra V, Chaudhry R, Dua T, et al. Association of Campylobacter jejuni infection with childhood Guillain-Barré syndrome: a case study. J Child Neurol 2009; 24(6):664–8.

25. Pope JE, Krizova A, Garg AX, et al. Campylobacter reactive arthritis: a systematic review. Semin Arthritis Rheum 2007;117:237–57.

26. Sanders JW, Frenck RW, Putnam SD, et al. Azithromycin and loperamide are comparable to levofloxacin and loperamide for the treatment of traveler's diarrhea in United States military personnel in Turkey. Clin Infect Dis 2007;45(3):294.

27. Tribble DR, Sanders JW, Pang LW, et al. Traveler's diarrhea in Thailand: randomized, double-blind trial comparing single-dose and 3 day azithromycin-based regimens with a 3-day levofloxacin regimen. Clin Infect Dis 2007;44(3):338.

28. Centers for Disease Control and Prevention. Biggest threats. Available at: http://www.cdc.gov/drugresistance/biggest_threats.html. Accessed June 8, 2016.

29. Majowicz SE, Musto J, Scallon E, et al. The global burden of nontyphoidal Salmonella gastroenteritis. Clin Infect Dis 2010;50(6):882–9.

30. Buchwald DS, Blaser MJ. A review of human salmonellosis: II. Duration of excretion following infection with nontyphi Salmonella. Rev Infect Dis 1984;6(3):345.

31. Gill CJ, Keene WE, Mohle-Boetani JC, et al. Alfalfa seed decontamination in a Salmonella outbreak. Emerg Infect Dis 2003;9(4):474–9.

32. Centers for Disease Control and Prevention. Outbreak of Salmonella enteritidis infection associated with consumption of raw egg shells, 1991. MMWR Morb Mortal Wkly Rep 1992;41(21):369–72.

33. Hennessy TW, Hedberg CW, Slutsker L, et al. A national outbreak of Salmonella enteritidis infections from ice cream. N Engl J Med 1996;334:1281–6.

34. Kimura AC, Reddy V, Marcus R, et al. Chicken consumption is a newly identified risk factor for sporadic salmonella enterica serotype enteritidis infections in the

United States: a case-control study in FoodNet sites. Clin Infect Dis 2004; 38(Suppl 3):S244–52.

35. Ao TT, Feasey NA, Gordon MA, et al. Global burden of invasive nontyphoidal Salmonella disease, 2010. Emerg Infect Dis 2015;21(6):941–9.

36. Burnett MW, Bass JW, Cook BA. Etiology of osteomyelitits complicating sickle cell disease. Pediatrics 1998;101(2):296–7.

37. Acheson D, Hohmann EL. Nontyphoidal salmenollosis. Clin Infect Dis 2001; 32(2):263–9.

38. Newton AE, Routh JA, Mahon BE. Typhoid & paratyphoid fever. In: CDC yellow book 2015. Available at: http://wwwnc.cdc.gov/travel/yellowbook/2016/infectious-diseases-related-to-travel/typhoid-paratyphoid-fever. Accessed June 20, 2016.

39. Angulo FJ, Tippen S, Sharp DJ, et al. A community waterborne outbreak of salmonellosis and the effectiveness of a boil water order. Am J Public Health 1997;87(4):580–4.

40. Parry CM, Hien TT, Dougan G, et al. Typhoid fever. N Engl J Med 2002;347(2): 1770–82.

41. Hatta M, Smits HL. Detection of Salmonella typhi by nested polymerase chain reaction in blood, urine, and stool samples. Am J Trop Med Hyg 2007;76(1): 139–43.

42. Crump JA, Luby SP, Mintz ED. The global burden of typhoid fever. Bull World Health Organ 2004;82(5):346–53.

43. Dupont HL, Levine MM, Hornick RB, et al. Inoculum size in shigellosis and implications for expected mode of transmission. J Infect Dis 1989;159(6):1126–8.

44. Kothary MH, Babu US. Infective dose of foodborne pathogens in volunteers: a review. J Food Saf 2001;21(1):49–68.

45. Scallan E, Hoekstra RM, Angulo FJ, et al. Foodborne illness acquired in the United Sates—major pathogens. Emerg Infect Dis 2011;17(1):7–15.

46. Baker KS, Dallman TJ, Ashton PM, et al. Intercontinental dissemination of azithromycin-resistant shigellosis through sexual transmission: a cross-sectional study. Lancet Infect Dis 2015;15(8):913–21.

47. DuPont HL, Hornick RB, Dawkins AT, et al. The response of a man to virulent Shigella flexneri 2a. J Infect Dis 1969;119(3):296–9.

48. von Seidlein L, Kim DR, Ali M, et al. A multicenter study of Shigella diarrhea in six Asian countries: disease burden, clinical manifestations, and microbiology. PLoS Med 2006;3(9):e353.

49. Stoll BJ, Glass MI, Huq MU, et al. Epidemiologic and clinical features of patients infected with Shigella who attended a diarrheal disease hospital in Bangladesh. J Infect Dis 1982;146(2):177–83.

50. Echeverria P, Sethabutr O, Pitarangsi C. Microbiology and diagnosis of infections with Shigella and enteroinvasive Escherichia coli. Rev Infect Dis 1991; 13(Suppl 4):S220–5.

51. Avital A, Maayan C, Goitein KJ. Incidence of convulsions and encephalopathy in childhood Shigella infections. Survey of 117 hospitalized patients. Clin Pediatr (Phila) 1982;21(11):645–8.

52. Khan WA, Dhar U, Salam MA, et al. Central nervous system manifestations of childhood shigellosis: prevalence, risk factors, and outcome. Pediatrics 1999; 103(2):E18.

53. Struelens MJ, Patte D, Kabir I, et al. Shigella septicemia: prevalence, presentation, risk factors, and outcome. J Infect Dis 1985;152(4):784–90.

54. Anjene AN, Fischer Walker CL, Black RE. Enteric pathogens and reactive arthritis: a systematic review of Campylobacter, salmonella, and Shigella-associated reactive arthritis. J Health Popul Nutr 2013;31(3):299–307.
55. Rahman M, Shoma S, Rashid H, et al. Increasing spectrum in antimicrobial resistance of Shigella isolates in Bangladesh: resistance to azithromycin and ceftriaxone and decreasing susceptibility to ciprofloxacin. J Health Popul Nutr 2007;25(2):158–67.
56. Karch H. The role of virulence factors in enterohemorrhagic Escherichia coli (EHEC)-associated hemolytic-uremic syndrome. Semin Thromb Hemost 2001; 27:207–13.
57. Picard C, Burley S, Bornet C, et al. Pathophysiology and treatment of typical and atypical hemolytic uremic syndrome. Pathol Biol (Paris) 2015;63(3):136–43.
58. Nathanson S, Kwon T, Elmaleh M, et al. Acute neurological involvement in diarrhea-associated hemolytic uremic syndrome. Clin J Am Soc Nephrol 2010;5(7):1218–28.
59. Edelman R, Karmali MA, Fleming PA. Summary of the international symposium and workshop on infections due to Verocytotoxin (Shiga-like-toxin)-producing Escherichia coli. J Infect Dis 1988;157(5):1102–4.
60. Centers for Disease Control and Prevention. Outbreak of Escherichia coli O104:H4 infections associated with sprout consumption—Europe and North America, May-July 2011. MMWR Morb Mortal Wkly Rep 2013;62(50):1029–31.
61. Grant J, Wendelboe AM, Wendel A, et al. Spinach-associated Escherichia coli O157:H7, Utah and Mexico, 2006. Emerg Infect Dis 2008;14(10):1633–6.
62. Bopp DJ, Sauders BD, Waring AL, et al. Detection, isolation, and molecular sub-typing of Escherichia coli O157:H7 and Campylobacter jejuni associated with a large waterborne outbreak. J Clin Microbiol 2003;41(10):174–80.
63. Riley LW, Remis RS, Helgerson SD, et al. Hemorrhagic colitis associated with a rare Escherichia coli serotype. N Engl J Med 1983;308:681–5.
64. Chen J, Griffiths MW. Cloning and sequencing of the gene encoding universal stress protein from Escherichia coli O157:H7 isolated from Jack-in-a-Box outbreak. Lett Appl Microbiol 1999;29(2):103–7.
65. Thorpe CM. Shiga toxin—producing Escherichia coli infection. Clin Infect Dis 2004;38(9):1298–303.
66. Rahal EA, Fadlallah SM, Nassar FJ, et al. Approaches to treatment of emerging Shiga toxin-producing Escherichia coli infections highlighting the O104:H4 sero-type. Front Cell Infect Microbiol 2015;5:24.
67. Feng Y, Xiao L. Zoonotic potential and molecular epidemiology of Giardia species and giardiasis. Clin Microbiol Rev 2011;24(1):110–40.
68. Baldursson S, Karanis P. Waterborne transmission of protozoan parasites: review of worldwide outbreaks – an update 2004-2010. Water Res 2011;45: 6603–14.
69. Painter JE, Gargano JW, Collier SA, et al. Giardiasis surveillance – United States, 2011-2012. MMWR Surveill Summ 2015;64(3):15–25.
70. Shaw PK, Brodsky RE, Lyman DO, et al. A communitywide outbreak of giardiasis with evidence of transmission by a municipal water supply. Ann Intern Med 1977;87(4):426–32.
71. Beer KD, Gargano JW, Roberts VA, et al. Surveillance for waterborne disease outbreaks associated with drinking water – United States, 2011-2012. MMWR Morb Mortal Wkly Rep 2015;64(31):842–8.

72. Beer KD, Gargano JW, Roberts VA, et al. Outbreaks associated with environmental and undetermined water exposures – United States, 2011-2012. MMWR Morb Mortal Wkly Rep 2015;64(31):849–51.

73. Hlavsa MC, Roberts VA, Kahler AM, et al. Outbreaks of illness associated with recreational water – United States, 2011-2012. MMWR Morb Mortal Wkly Rep 2015;64(24):668–72.

74. Mintz ED, Hudson-Wragg M, Mshar P, et al. Foodborne giardiasis in a corporate office setting. J Infect Dis 1993;167(1):250–3.

75. Quick R, Paugh K, Addiss D, et al. Restaurant-associated outbreak of giardiasis. J Infect Dis 1992;166(3):673–6.

76. Esch KJ, Petersen CA. Transmission and epidemiology of zoonotic protozoal disease of companion animals. Clin Microbiol Rev 2013;26(1):58–85.

77. Thompson RCA. The zoonotic significance and molecular epidemiology of Giardia and giardiasis. Vet Parasitol 2004;126:15–35.

78. Chute CG, Smith RP, Baron JA. Risk factors for endemic giardiasis. Am J Public Health 1987;77(5):585–7.

79. Stuart JM, Orr HJ, Warburton FG, et al. Risk factors for sporadic giardiasis: a case-control study in southwestern England. Emerg Infect Dis 2003;9(2):229–33.

80. Ekdahl K, Andersson Y. Imported giardiasis: impact of international travel, immigration, and adoption. Am J Trop Med Hyg 2005;72(6):825–30.

81. Hill DR. Giardiasis: issues in diagnosis and management. Infect Dis Clin North Am 1993;7(3):503–25.

82. Chester AC, Macmurray FG, Restifo MD, et al. Giardiasis as a chronic disease. Dig Dis Sci 1985;30(3):215–8.

83. Stark D, Barratt JLN, van Hal S, et al. Clinical significance of enteric protozoa in the immunosuppressed human population. Clin Microbiol Rev 2009;22(4):634–50.

84. Lengerich EJ, Addiss DG, Juranek DD. Severe giardiasis in the United States. Clin Infect Dis 1994;18(5):760–3.

85. Farthing MJ, Mata L, Urrutia JJ, et al. Natural history of Giardia infection on infants and children in rural Guatemala and its impact on physical growth. Am J Clin Nutr 1986;43(3):395–405.

86. Berkman DS, Lescano AG, Gilman RH, et al. Effects of stunting, diarrhoeal disease, and parasitic infection during infancy on cognition in late childhood: a follow-up study. Lancet 2002;359:564–71.

87. Welsh JD, Poley JR, Hensley J, et al. Intestinal disaccharidase and alkaline phosphatase activity in giardiasis. J Pediatr Gastroenterol Nutr 1984;3:37–40.

88. Heyworth MF. Diagnostic testing for Giardia infections. Trans R Soc Trop Med Hyg 2014;108(3):123–5.

89. Garcia LS, Shimizu RY. Evaluation of nine immunoassay kits (enzyme immunoassay and direct fluorescence) for detection of Giardia lamblia and Cryptosporidium parvum in human fecal specimens. J Clin Microbiol 1997;35(6):1526–9.

90. Rossignol JF. Cryptosporidium and Giardia: treatment options and prospects for new drugs. Exp Parasitol 2010;124:45–53.

91. Gardner TB, Hill DR. Treatment of giardiasis. Clin Microbiol Rev 2001;14(1):114–28.

92. Huang DB, Clinton White A. An updated review on cryptosporidium and giardia. Gastroenterol Clin North Am 2006;35:291–314.

93. Navin TR. Cryptosporidiosis in humans: review of recent epidemiologic studies. Eur J Epidemiol 1985;1(2):77–83.

94. Painter JE, Hlava MC, Collier SA, et al. Cryptosporidiosis surveillance – United States, 2011-2012. MMWR Surveill Summ 2015;64(3):1–13.
95. Yoder JS, Harral C, Beach MJ. Cryptosporidiosis surveillance – United States, 2006-2008. MMWR Surveill Summ 2010;59:1–14.
96. MacKenzie WR, Schell WL, Blair KA, et al. Massive outbreak of waterborne cryptosporidium infection in Milwaukee, Wisconsin: recurrent of illness and risk of secondary transmission. Clin Infect Dis 1995;21(1):57–62.
97. Fayer R. Cryptosporidium: a water-borne zoonotic parasite. Vet Parasitol 2004; 126:37–56.
98. Sorvillo FJ, Fujoka K, Nahlen B, et al. Swimming-associated cryptosporidiosis. Am J Public Health 1992;82:742–4.
99. Millard PS, Gensheimer KF, Addiss DG, et al. An outbreak of cryptosporidiosis from fresh-pressed apple cider. JAMA 1994;272:1592–6.
100. Roy SL, DeLong SM, Stenzel SA. Risk factors for sporadic cryptosporidiosis among immunocompetent persons in the United States from 1999 to 2001. J Clin Microbiol 2004;42(7):2944–51.
101. Goh S, Reacher M, Casemore DP, et al. Sporadic cryptosporidiosis, North Cumbria, England, 1996-2000. Emerg Infect Dis 2004;10(6):1007–15.
102. Lendner M, Daugschies A. Cryptosporidium infections: molecular advances. Parasitology 2014;141(11):1511–32.
103. Hunter PR, Nichols G. Epidemiology and clinical features of Cryptosporidium infection in immunocompromised patients. Clin Microbiol Rev 2002;15:145–54.
104. Vakil NB, Schwartz SM, Buggy BP, et al. Biliary cryptosporidiosis in HIV-infected people after the waterborne outbreak of cryptosporidiosis in Milwaukee. N Engl J Med 1996;334:19–23.
105. Hojlyng N, Jensen BN. Respiratory cryptosporidiosis in HIV-positive patients. Lancet 1988;1(8585):590–1.
106. Arrowood MJ, Sterling CR. Comparison of conventional staining methods and monoclonal antibody-based methods for Cryptosporidium oocyst detection. J Clin Microbiol 1989;27:1490–5.
107. Van Lint P, Rossen JW, Vermeiren S, et al. Detection of Giardia lamblia, Cryptosporidium spp. and Entamoeba histolytica in clinical stool samples by using multiplex real-time PCR after automated DNA isolation. Acta Clin Belg 2013; 68:188–92.
108. Rossignol JF, Ayoub A, Ayers MS. Treatment of diarrhea caused by Cryptosporidium parvum: a prospective randomized, double-blind, placebo-controlled study of nitazoxanide. J Infect Dis 2001;184(1):103–6.
109. Abubakar I, Aliyu SH, Arumugam C, et al. Treatment of cryptosporidiosis in immunocompromised individuals: systematic review and meta-analysis. Br J Clin Pharmacol 2007;63(4):387–93.

Tickborne Infections

Kathleen M. Barta, PA-C, MPAS

KEYWORDS

- Tickborne infections • Lyme disease • Ehrlichia • Anaplasma • Babesiosis
- Rocky Mountain spotted fever

KEY POINTS

- Tickborne infections are increasing throughout the United States, and diagnosis can be missed if appropriate history and physical examination are not done.
- Appropriate testing is essential for diagnosis of most tickborne infections.
- Empiric therapy with appropriate antibiotics should not be delayed if patient is ill and suspicion for tickborne infection is high.
- Patients do not always remember a tick bite. This should not influence testing and treatment if history is concerning for tickborne infection.

INTRODUCTION

Tickborne diseases are found throughout the United States and the world, and can be caused by bacteria, viruses, or parasites. Many tickborne illnesses, including Lyme disease, *Ehrlichia*, and anaplasmosis, are increasing owing to improved diagnostic methods, increasing human population, and the sprawl of habitation into previously rural areas. Tickborne diseases are serious health problems affecting hundreds of thousands of people in the United States each year.[1] From 2013 to 2016, the Centers for Disease Control and Prevention has increased the number of reported Lyme cases in the United States from 30,000 to 300,000; a 10-fold increase.[1]

Diagnosing a tickborne illness can be challenging, because symptoms are often vague, like headache, fever, and malaise, which can mimic other illnesses. Many patients do not remember a tick bite or rash, and travel history is not always obtained by the clinician, leading to a delay in treatment and increase in morbidity and mortality.

This article concentrates on the most common tickborne diseases affecting the United States today—Lyme disease, *ehrlichiosis and anaplasmosis*, babesiosis, and Rocky Mountain spotted fever (RMSF). New tickborne diseases, such as Powassan disease, heartland virus, and southern tick-associated rash illness are emerging and research is ongoing. Previous well-circumscribed boundaries for endemic tick areas are changing as our population grows and our environment changes. Clinicians face

The author has nothing to disclose.
Infectious Diseases Specialists of Southeastern Wisconsin, 150 South Sunnyslope Road, Suite 136, Brookfield, WI 53005, USA
E-mail address: kbarta@idisease.com

Physician Assist Clin 2 (2017) 247–260
http://dx.doi.org/10.1016/j.cpha.2016.12.007
2405-7991/17/© 2016 Elsevier Inc. All rights reserved.

the challenge of diagnosing and treating regional tickborne illnesses, but also keeping current with updates and emerging infections.

LYME DISEASE

Lyme disease is a bacterial infection, caused by the spirochete *Borrelia burgdorferi*, and transmitted by the black legged or deer tick (*Ixodes scapularis*). It is the most common tickborne infection in the United States, with about 300,000 cases diagnosed annually.[1,2] Lyme disease is most commonly reported in New England, mid-Atlantic states, and north central United States. Less commonly, it is found in the western United States, where it is transmitted by the western blacklegged tick, *Ixodes pacificus*. Of interest, although Lyme disease has been reported in 48 states, data suggest that cases are concentrated in 13 states (Connecticut, Delaware, Maine, Maryland, Massachusetts, Minnesota, New Hampshire, New Jersey, New York, Pennsylvania, Vermont, Virginia and Wisconsin), with the highest incidence annually in Pennsylvania.[1]

Lyme disease occurs throughout Europe, where it is caused by *Borrelia afzelii* and *Borrelia garinii*, and transmitted by the sheep tick *Ixodes ricinus*.[3] The *I scapularis* tick may also transmit *Anaplasma phagocytophilum*, which causes human granulocytic anaplasmosis (previously called ehrlichia) and/or *Babesia microti*, which causes babesiosis.[4] A bite from an infected tick may lead to any of these infections or, less frequently, coinfection. The most common reservoirs for *B burgdorferi* are white-tailed deer, mice, chipmunks, birds, and other small mammals. Mosquitoes are not vectors for Lyme disease.

Etiology

Most cases of early Lyme disease occur during spring and summer when ticks are feeding, but tick bites can occur throughout the year. Most often, disease is transmitted by ticks in the nymphal stage, although female adult ticks can transmit bacteria as well. Although the nymphal I. scapularis tick is more likely to be infected with B burgdorferi, adult ticks are larger and are likely to be noticed and removed more quickly (Fig. 1). It takes at least 2 hours for ticks to attach to the skin, and the most common attachment sites are legs, back, groin, axilla, and waist.[3] In children, the head, scalp, and neck are frequent sites of tick bites. *B burgdorferi* bacteria lives in the midgut of ticks, and must replicate and migrate to the salivary glands to be transmitted with the tick bite.[3] For this reason, it takes 36 to 48 hours after the tick attaches to be infected with *B burgdorferi*. Lyme disease cannot be transmitted from person to person.[1] Dogs and cats can become infected from a tick bite, but there is no evidence that they transmit Lyme disease to humans, although if a tick is present it can move to a human host.

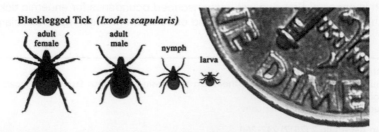

Fig. 1. Blacklegged tick life stages. (*Courtesy of* the Centers for Disease Control and Prevention.)

Clinical Manifestations

Lyme disease is divided into 3 stages: early localized, early disseminated, and late stage infection. Most patients do not exhibit all stages, and stages may blend together. Lyme disease primarily affects the skin, heart, nervous system, and joints.

Early Localized Infection

Early localized Lyme disease is cutaneous, and manifested by erythema migrans (EM). EM has been estimated to be present in anywhere from 60% to 80% of infected patients, and begins at the site of the tick bite between 3 and 32 days later, although 7 to 14 days seems to be most common.[3,5] Typically described as a bull's eye or target lesion, lesions can be confluent, patchy, and have central clearing or necrosis. Diagnosis can be made by clinical examination alone, although lesions must be at least 5 cm in diameter, and in patients living in or traveling to an endemic area.[1,5,6] Multiple, often smaller skin lesions are consistent with early disseminated Lyme infection owing to hematogenous seeding. Different genotypic strains of bacteria may increase risk of disseminated infection (Fig. 2).[3,7]

EM differential includes Southern tick-associated rash, which is transmitted by *Amblyomma americanum* tick. There is some overlap in the geographic areas, primarily in the mid-central and southeastern United States. However, unless there is positive identification of the *A americanum* tick, patients in endemic Lyme areas should be presumed to have Lyme disease and treated with appropriate antibiotics.[7]

Not all patients with early Lyme disease present with EM lesions. Other early symptoms include intermittent fevers, chills, diffuse myalgias, arthralgias, fatigue, headache, lymphadenopathy, and weakness. Extracutaneous signs of infection include neurologic conditions, such as cranial nerve palsy, meningitis, and carditis, which typically presents as atrioventricular block or less commonly as myopericarditis.

Early Disseminated Infection

Multiple EM lesions are seen in early disseminated infection owing to spirochetemia. These typically develop a few days after the initial EM lesion in 45% to 50% of patients, and are unrelated to size or duration of EM lesions.[5,6]

Approximately 60% of patients with EM who are not treated will go on to have a monoarticular or oligoarticular arthritis, typically involving the knee; approximately

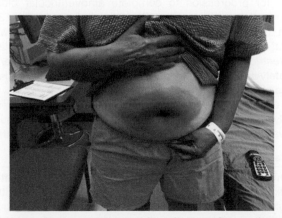

Fig. 2. Erythema migrans lesion in patient with early Lyme disease. (*Courtesy of* D. Letzer, DO, Brookfield, WI.)

10% to 15% will have a neurologic manifestation, the most common of which is facial nerve palsy, and approximately 5% will have a cardiac complication, usually varying degrees of atrioventricular block.[5]

Neurologic Disease

Untreated Lyme disease can cause both acute and chronic neurologic changes. Approximately 15% to 20% of untreated patients will have some degree of neurologic involvement, typically 2 to 8 weeks after the onset of disease.[5,8] Cranial nerve palsy, lymphocytic meningitis, acute radiculopathy, and peripheral neuritis can all be seen alone or in combination, although facial palsy and meningitis are most common. Cranial nerve involvement owing to Lyme disease typically occurs early and abruptly in the course of illness, with involvement of cranial nerve VII being most common.[9]

Symptoms depend on the area of the nervous system involved, with headache, fever, and stiff neck typically seen in meningitis patients. Patients with cranial nerve palsy may have either unilateral or bilateral facial palsy. Because bilateral facial nerve palsy is uncommon, patients presenting with these findings from an endemic Lyme area should be screened for Lyme disease.[9] Encephalomyelitis is less commonly seen, and patients may exhibit fevers, confusion, difficulty concentrating, and emotional lability.[5,9]

Lumbar puncture is indicated if neurologic involvement is seen. Cerebrospinal fluid (CSF) will show pleocytosis, elevated protein concentration, and low to normal glucose concentrations.[2] Central nervous system involvement can also be demonstrated by intrathecal borrelial antibody production, although this test is not readily available and has poor sensitivity.[7] Encephalomyelitis diagnosis must be confirmed by antibody production against *B burgdorferi* in the CSF, with a higher titer of antibody in CSF than in serum. Abnormalities seen in the CSF respond quickly to appropriate antibiotic administration.[2]

Lyme Carditis

Carditis is a rare complication of Lyme disease, and occurs in 0.5% to 10.0% of cases in Europe and North America.[10] Atrioventricular heart block is the most common cardiac manifestation of untreated Lyme disease, starting several weeks to several months after tick bite. Although third-degree heart block is typically the most common, progression from first-degree to third-degree heart block can occur within minutes.[9,10] The greatest risk for progression to complete atrioventricular block, which may develop rapidly, occurs in patients with a PR interval of greater than 30 ms. Because Lyme carditis can be life threatening, patients who are symptomatic with palpitations, syncope, dyspnea, have second-degree or third-degree atrioventricular block, or have first degree atrioventricular block with a PR interval of 30 ms or greater should be hospitalized immediately and started on telemetry. Treatment for Lyme disease with intravenous antibiotics should be started immediately.

Other cardiac complications include pericarditis, myocarditis, ventricular tachycardia, and (rarely) dilated cardiomyopathy.[5] Severe congestive heart failure or the development of valvular heart disease is not associated typically with Lyme disease.

Late Lyme Disease

Lyme arthritis, which occurs weeks to months (average 6 months) after a tick bite, is considered a hallmark of late Lyme disease.[8] It is typically intermittent, migratory, monoarticular or pauciarticular, and most often affects the knee joint. Knee effusions, Baker's cysts, erythema, and pain are reported commonly. Lyme arthritis occurs in fewer than 10% of patients.[4] This is likely owing to increased awareness of Lyme disease, and earlier treatment. Confirmation of diagnosis must be made by serologic testing. Aspiration of synovial fluid will show mild inflammation, with a median leukocyte count of 24,250 leukocytes/mm^3 and a granulocytic predominance.[4] Positive polymerase chain reaction (PCR) testing of the synovial fluid confirms the diagnosis only in a seropositive patient. A seronegative patient with positive PCR in a joint fluid specimen should not be considered to have Lyme disease. Other late manifestations of Lyme disease include encephalopathy, encephalomyelitis, and peripheral neuropathy.[4]

Diagnosis

The standard laboratory method for diagnosing Lyme disease is detection of antibodies to B burgdorferi. A 2-tiered system is currently standard of care in the United States.[11] The first tier is a quantitative enzyme immunoassay to detect antibodies against B burgdorferi. If this is negative, no further testing is needed. If this test is positive or equivocal, a second-tier test, Western blotting, should be done; immunoglobulin (Ig)M and IgG immunoblots if early disease is suspected ($\leq$4 weeks since tick bite) and IgG alone if late disease is suspected (>4 weeks since tick bite). At least 2 IgM bands must be positive in early disease, and at least 5 IgG bands must be positive in mid or late stage disease.[7]

If a patient presents with an EM lesion and resides in or has traveled to an endemic area, diagnosis is based on clinical examination findings alone. No serologic testing is needed, and treatment should be initiated with appropriate antibiotics. Of note, current serologic testing in early Lyme disease has sensitivity of less than 50% in early disease.[12] In addition, after antibodies develop in Lyme disease, they may persist for many years, leading to confusion in the serologic interpretation of active infection and treatment response.

Treatment

All recommended antibiotics and their corresponding doses are based on Infectious Disease Society of America guidelines.[4]

- Early Lyme disease, with or without EM lesions, and without complications: Adult therapy: Doxycycline 100 mg orally twice daily for 14 days. Alternative therapy for patients allergic to doxycycline or pregnant women: amoxicillin 500 mg orally, 3 times daily or cefuroxime axetil 500 mg orally twice daily for 14 days.
  Pediatric therapy: for children less than 8 years old, amoxicillin 50 mg/kg per day in 3 divided doses (maximum 500 mg per dose) or cefuroxime axetil 30 mg/kg per day in 2 divided doses (maximum of 500 mg per dose). If the patient is 8 years of age or younger, doxycycline 4 mg/kg per day (maximum of 100 mg per dose) in 2 divided doses may be used. Duration of therapy remains 14 days for children.
  First-generation cephalosporins are not an effective treatment for Lyme disease.
- Lyme meningitis and other early neurologic disease should be treated with intravenous antibiotics:
  o Ceftriaxone, 2 g once per day intravenously for 14 to 28 days. Alternatives are cefotaxime, 2 g intravenously every 8 hours, or penicillin G, 18 to 24 million units intravenously per day, divided into doses every 4 hours. Note, dosing is based on normal renal function.
  o Doxycycline 100 to 200 mg orally twice daily for 14 to 28 days can be used in patients who are allergic to beta-lactam antibiotics.[4] Doxycycline has excellent oral absorption, so intravenous formulation is not needed.[4]
  o Ceftriaxone 50 to 75 mg/kg daily can be used in children (maximum of 2 g per day). Cefotaxime 150 to 200 mg/kg daily divided into 3 doses (maximum of

6 g per day) or penicillin G 200,000 to 400,000 units/kg daily, given every 4 hours (maximum of 18–24 million units per day) are alternatives to ceftriaxone.
   ○ Children greater than 8 years of age can also be treated with oral doxycycline, 100 mg twice daily for 14 to 28 days.
 • Patients with atrioventricular heart block or myopericarditis associated with Lyme disease should be hospitalized and monitored with continuous telemetry. Antibiotic treatment with ceftriaxone, 2 g intravenously daily, should be given while the patient is hospitalized.[4] Oral antibiotic therapy with doxycycline, 100 mg twice daily, may be used upon hospital discharge or when advanced heart block resolves.[3,4] Duration of therapy is 14 to 21 days.
 • Lyme arthritis can be treated with oral or intravenous antibiotics.[4] Doxycyline, or alternative regimens with amoxicillin or cefuroxime axetil, as outlined in Early Lyme Disease Treatment, should be given for 28 days. If patients have concomitant neurologic symptoms, therapy with ceftriaxone, 2 g intravenously daily for 28 days should be given.
 • Patients with persistent or recurrent joint swelling after an initial course of antibiotics should be given an additional 28 days of oral antibiotics, or 14 to 28 days of parenteral antibiotics. If patients have no resolution of arthritis despite intravenous therapy, and if PCR results of synovial fluid or tissue culture are negative, symptomatic treatment with a nonsteroidal antiinflammatory agent is recommended.[4] Pediatric patients younger than 8 years of age should be treated with oral therapy, as outlined in Early Lyme Disease Treatment, for 28 days (Table 1).

Prevention

Currently, the best method for preventing Lyme disease is to avoid a tick bite. This strategy includes avoiding tick-infested areas, wearing protective clothing, tucking the shirt into pants and tucking the pants into socks or boots, using tick repellant with DEET, and checking the entire body for ticks daily with prompt removal of an attached tick if residing or traveling in an endemic area. Shower as soon as possible after being outdoors in endemic areas. If a tick is found, remove gently with fine tipped tweezer, avoiding a twisting motion to prevent breaking tick apart. Clean area with alcohol after.

If a tick bite occurs, a single 200-mg dose of doxycycline for adults, or 4 mg/kg to a child 8 years of age or older can be given within 72 hours of the time the tick was removed. It is recommended for areas where the local rate of infection of ticks with B burgdorferi is 20% or greater.[4] Amoxicillin and cephalosporins are not recommended for prophylaxis owing to lack of data supporting their use. Pregnant women and children younger than age 8 should be screened for Lyme disease following guidelines as stated, and treated if there is documented positive serology.[4] Currently, no vaccine is available.

HUMAN BABESIOSIS
Etiology

Babesiosis is a zoonotic infection caused by intraerythrocytic protozoa and transmitted by ticks. The first documented human case occurred in a splenectomized patient in Croatia who died after an acute febrile illness.[13] The first case of babesiosis in an immunocompetent patient was found in Massachusetts in 1969.[13] The agent was Babesia microti, and the tick vector was Ixodes dammini, now Ixodes scapularis.[13,14]

There are more than 100 species of babesia, but only a few infect humans. The majority of cases in the United States are caused by B microti and occur primarily from

Table 1
Lyme disease treatment

Condition	Antibiotic	Duration	Comments
Early Lyme disease/erythema migrans	*Doxycycline* 100 mg twice daily Pediatric: 4 mg/kg/d Divided into 2 doses, maximum of 100 mg/dose *Amoxicillin* 500 mg 3 times daily Pediatric: 50 mg/kg/d Divided into 3 doses, maximum of 500 mg/dose *Cefuroxime axetil*, 500 mg twice daily Pediatric: 30 mg/kg/d, maximum of 500 mg/dose Divided into 2 doses	14 d	Doxycycline for use in patients > age 8 and nonpregnant women
Meningitis	*Ceftriaxone* 2 g IV daily Pediatric: 50–75 mg/kg daily – maximum of 2 g/d *Penicillin G* 18–24 million units, every 4 h *Doxycycline* 200–400 mg Divided into 2 doses daily Pediatric: >8 y of age 4–8 mg/kg/d in 2 divided doses, maximum of 100 mg/dose	14–28 d	For patients intolerant of Beta-lactams, >8 y os age and nonpregnant women. Good oral absorption; do not need IV administration.
Cranial nerve palsy without meningitis	If patient has normal CSF examination, no signs of meningitis, treat with same regimen for early Lyme disease. If patient has clinical and laboratory evidence of CNS Involvement, treat with same regimen for Lyme meningitis.	—	—

Late Lyme disease	Lyme arthritis
	  Doxycycline 100 mg twice daily
	  Pediatric: 4 mg/kg/d
	  Divided into 2 doses, maximum of 100 mg/dose
	  Amoxicillin 500 mg 3 times daily
	  Pediatric: 50 mg/kg/d
	  Divided into 3 doses, maximum of 500 mg/dose
	  Cefuroxime axetil, 500 mg 2 twice daily
	  Pediatric: 30 mg/kg/d
	  Divided into 2 doses, maximum of 500 mg/dose
	Late Lyme neurologic disease
	  Adult patients with neurologic disease should receive IV antibiotics with ceftriaxone, cefotaxime or penicillin G. See Lyme meningitis for dosing and duration.
		28 d	If persistent or recurrent joint swelling after 28 d, retreat with another 4-wk course of oral antibiotics or 2–4 wk of IV antibiotics.

(*continued on next page*)

Table 1 (*continued*)			
Condition	Antibiotic	Duration	Comments
Lyme carditis	*Ceftriaxone* 2 g IV daily Pediatric: 50–75 mg/kg daily, maximum of 2 g/d *Penicillin G* 18–24 million units, every 4 h *Doxycycline* 200–400 mg Divided into 2 doses daily Pediatric: >8 y of age 4–8 mg/kg/d in 2 divided doses, maximum of 100 mg/dose	14–21 d	IV antibiotic recommended for hospitalized patients. Patients can be discharged on oral antibiotics for completion of therapy.

Abbreviations: CNS, central nervous system; CSF, cerebrospinal fluid; IV, intravenous.

spring to early fall. Geographic locations roughly correspond with those of Lyme disease, and are most prevalent in the Northeast and upper Midwest regions, although the West coast and Southeastern United States have reported a few cases with *B duncani* and *B divergens*.[13]

B microti is transmitted by the *I scapularis* tick, the same tick that transmits *B burgdorferi* and *A phagocytophilum*, and the primary vector is the white footed mouse (*Peromyscus leucopus*).[13–15] Larval ticks feed on infected mice in late summer and the mice retain the parasite in multiple stages until the following year. The disease is transmitted to vertebrate hosts when the nymphal tick feeds the following summer. Ticks feed on the white tailed deer, and it is thought that the enlarging deer population, along with close human proximity, has been partially responsible for the increase in human babesiosis.

There have been documented cases of babesiosis through blood transfusion, and many cases have been severe, because transfusion recipients are frequently ill or immunosuppressed.[13] There are no Babesia screening tests for blood donors at this time.

Clinical Manifestations

Clinical features of babesiosis range from subclinical to severe and can mimic those of malaria. Patients become ill 1 to 4 weeks after the bite of an infected tick or up to 9 weeks after receiving a blood transfusion from an infected patient. Patients may present with fevers, severe rigors, fatigue, headache, myalgias, arthralgias, nausea, and anorexia. Significant laboratory findings include thrombocytopenia, hemolytic anemia, and elevated liver enzymes.[7] Patients over the age of 50, and those with human immunodeficiency virus infection, malignancy, asplenia, or other immune-compromising illnesses are at increased risk of severe disease. Severe cases can be associated with marked thrombocytopenia, disseminated intravascular coagulation, hemodynamic instability, acute respiratory distress, renal failure, hepatic compromise, altered mental status, and death.[1]

Diagnosis

A definitive diagnosis of babesiosis should be made by microscopic examination of thin blood smears (Wright or Giemsa staining under oil immersion). Thick blood smears are not recommended, because babesial parasites may be too small to be visualized.[15] PCR testing can be useful in early disease and convalescent testing, when parasitemia is low, making parasites difficult to see on thin blood smear. Serology (IgG and IgM antibody testing) can confirm diagnosis of babesiosis, but it is not reliable, because the antibody may be undetectable early in the course of disease and can persist after resolution of infection.[7]

Treatment

All recommended antibiotics and their corresponding doses are based on Infectious Disease Society of America guidelines.[4]

- Atovaquone, 750 mg every 12 hours plus azithromycin, 500 mg on day 1, then 250 mg daily for 7 days, is standard adult therapy.
- Clindamycin 600 mg every 8 hours and quinine, 650 mg every 8 hours is equally effective, but less well-tolerated and has greater side effects than atovaquone and azithromycin.
- For immunosuppressed patients, atovaquone, as described, plus a higher dose of azithromycin, 600 to 1000 mg/d, is recommended. The duration of therapy remains the same.
- For patients with severe babesiosis, intravenous clindamycin and quinine should be given. Longer duration of antibiotic therapy may be necessary until parasitemia clears.
- Pediatric therapy: atovaquone, 20 mg/kg every 12 hours (maximum of 750 mg/dose) plus azithromycin 10 mg/kg once on day 1 (maximum of 500 mg/dose) and 5 mg/kg (maximum of 250 mg/dose) orally daily thereafter for 7 days.
- Clindamycin 7 to 10 mg/kg intravenous or orally (maximum of 600 mg/dose) and quinine 8 mg/kg orally every 8 hours (maximum of 650 mg/dose) can be used as alternative for pediatric patients unable to tolerate or allergic to atovaquone and/or azithromycin.

All patients with active babesiosis should be treated with antimicrobial therapy owing to the risk of complications.[4] Symptomatic patients whose serum contains antibody to Babesia but have negative thin smear without identifiable parasites or are without babesial DNA by PCR should not receive treatment.[4] Treatment is not recommended for asymptomatic individuals.

Partial or complete red blood cell exchange transfusion is indicated for patients with high-grade parasitemia ($\geq$10%), or pulmonary, renal, or hepatic failure owing to illness.[4] Patients should be monitored closely with daily laboratory testing to follow hemoglobin and hematocrit, and a thin blood smear to evaluate parasite load. In patients with mild or moderate illness, symptoms generally improve within 48 hours and complete resolution of symptoms occurs by 3 months. Patients with severe illness may take much longer to recover and may have persistence of low-grade parasitemia for months after treatment.[4,7]

If patients have persistent or severe symptoms that do not improve despite appropriate antibiotic therapy, the possibility of coinfection with Lyme disease or human granulocytic anaplasmosis should be considered, and appropriate testing done.[4]

Prevention

Prevention of tick bite is the same as recommended for Lyme disease. Currently, there is no vaccine available.

ANAPLASMOSIS AND EHRLICHIOSIS

Ehrlichiosis is the common name for infections caused by intracellular gram-negative bacteria Anaplasma and *Ehrlichia*. Three species cause human tickborne infection in the United States. *Anaplasma phagocytophilum*, the agent of human granulocytic anaplasmosis, is transmitted by *Ixodes scapularis* (deer tick) in the eastern United States and the *Ixodes pacificus* (black legged tick) in the northwestern/Pacific coast region. *Ixodes* species ticks are the same vectors for *B burgdorferi* and *B microti*, and infections are found in the same endemic area. *Ehrlichia chaffeensis* causes human monocytic ehrlichiosis (HME) and *Ehrlichia ewingii* causes human ewingii ehrlichiosis. Both are transmitted by *Americanum amblyomma* (the Lone Star tick), which is endemic in the south and southeastern United States.

Etiology

When the tick vector takes a blood meal from a mammal, bacteria from tick saliva are injected into the host. Bacteria preferentially infect circulating leukocytes, causing a febrile illness. *E chafeensis* infects monocytes and macrophages. *A phagocytophilum* and *E ewingii* infect neutrophilic granulocytes. White tail deer are the principal reservoir for HME and the white footed mouse and white tail deer are the most common hosts for human granulocytic anaplasmosis. Transmission of bacteria occurs 24 to 48 hours after tick attachment. Most infections occur from April through October, and are reportable in the United States.[16] In addition, ehrlichiosis is transmittable through blood transfusion and also maternal–child transmission.[17]

Clinical Manifestations

Incubation period for HME typically is 1 to 2 weeks. Symptoms vary by patient and can include fatigue, myalgias, fevers, chills, malaise, weakness, nausea, and abdominal pain. Rash is not common, and when seen, coinfection with *B burgdorferi* or *Rickettsia rickettsii* in the appropriate setting should be considered. Symptoms are typically worse in an immunosuppressed patient (ie, infected with the human immunodeficiency virus, organ transplant recipients, cancer patients, or those undergoing chemotherapy), and those patients with HME can develop a septic shocklike syndrome.[16] Central nervous system symptoms are less common, but meningitis can occur. Complications include seizures, coma, and renal and respiratory failure. The most common laboratory findings are leukopenia (many times with a left shift), thrombocytopenia, and elevated liver transaminases. Anemia may also be seen.

Diagnosis

Laboratory testing by PCR can be used for both human granulocytic anaplasmosis and HME; however, sensitivity is low, and a negative result does not rule it out.[17] Antibodies may be negative in the first 7 to 10 days of illness. The gold standard serologic test for diagnosis of anaplasmosis and HME is the indirect immunofluorescence assay using *A phagocytophilum* antigen or *E chaffeensis* antigen, performed on paired serum samples to demonstrate a 4-fold increase in antibody titers.[17] The first sample should be taken the first week of illness and the second 2 to 4 weeks later. Concurrent testing for Lyme disease is recommended given the possibility of coinfection.

Treatment

All recommended antibiotics and their corresponding doses are based on Infectious Disease Society of America guidelines.[4]

- Doxycycline 100 mg twice daily for 10 to 14 days for adult patients.
- Doxycycline 4 mg/kg in 2 divided doses daily (maximum of 100 mg/dose) for children weighing less than 45 kg. If weighing more than 45 kg, the adult dose should be used.[a]
- Pregnant patients can be treated with doxycycline 100 mg twice daily for 10 to 14 days if symptomatic and/or severely ill. The alternative treatment is rifampin 300 mg twice daily.[18,b]

Prevention

Prevention of tick bite is the same as recommended for Lyme disease. Currently, there is no vaccine available.

ROCKY MOUNTAIN SPOTTED FEVER
Etiology

RMSF is a tickborne illness caused by *R rickettsii*, a small gram-negative bacillus. It is found throughout the United States, but primarily in North Carolina, Oklahoma, Arkansas, Tennessee, and Missouri.[1] In the eastern and south central United States, the principal vector is *Dermacentor variabilis* (the American dog tick). West of the Mississippi, *Dermacentor andersonii* (Rocky Mountain wood tick) is the common vector. *Rhipicephalus sanguineus* (the common brown dog tick) is also a vector for RMSF in the southwestern United States, and has been linked with severe infections on Indian reservations in Arizona.[20] The tick is both the vector and the main reservoir, and only adult ticks feed on humans. Rickettsiae are spread hematogenously after a tick has bitten and fed for 6 to 10 hours.[21] Infection can also occur by exposure to infected tick hemolymph during the removal of a tick from a person or domestic animals, particularly when the tick is crushed during removal.[22] Rickettsial infection is spread via lymphatics and small blood vessels to the systemic and pulmonary circulation. Rickettsiae preferentially attach to vascular endothelium, leading to vascular injury, causing cell destruction and affecting tissue and multiple organs.[22]

Clinical Manifestations

Fever, myalgia, and headache is the classic triad of symptoms associated with RMSF. The incubation period is usually 1 week, but can be anywhere from 3 to 12 days after tick bite. Nonpruritic, macular lesions typically present on the ankles an wrists, and then on the trunk, palms, and soles (Fig. 3).

These lesions may later hemorrhage and form petechiae. Rash is present in only 14% of patients on the first day of illness, and 49% during the first 3 days.[21,22] The extent of the rash does not correspond with the severity of illness. Other symptoms include malaise, nausea, vomiting, and abdominal pain. Untreated, RMSF can lead to congestive heart failure, arrhythmias, and central nervous system involvement with confusion and lethargy owing to encephalitis, ataxia, delirium, and seizures.[22] Severely ill patients can develop renal, respiratory, or hepatic failure leading to death. Common laboratory findings are anemia, thrombocytopenia, increased liver transaminase levels, and hyponatremia.

---

[a] Short course of doxycycline considered safe in children; lower risk of dental staining than tetracycline.[19]

[b] Rifampin will not cover *B burgdorferi*.

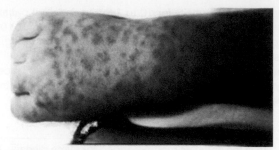

Fig. 3. Macular rash from Rocky Mountain spotted fever. (*Courtesy of* the Centers for Disease Control and Prevention.)

Diagnosis

Clinicians should not wait for laboratory confirmation of disease to begin therapy in patients with suspected RMSF based on clinical examination findings and history, owing to the potential severity of the disease. *R rickettsii* cannot be cultured in most laboratories. Antibodies to *R rickettsii* are detectable 7 to 10 days after onset of symptoms, and the optimal time to obtain convalescent titers is 14 to 21 days after illness onset. Serologic testing should be done to demonstrate a 4-fold change in antibody titers (IgG, IgM) using paired samples, with the first sample obtained at 1 week and the second sample 2 to 4 weeks later.[19]

Treatment

All recommended antibiotics and their corresponding doses are based on Centers for Disease Control guidelines.[19]

- Doxycycline 100 mg twice daily, either orally or intravenously for adult patients. Treatment should be continued for 3 days after patient has become afebrile (the minimum duration of therapy is 5–7 days).
- Doxycycline 4 mg/kg in 2 divided doses daily (maximum of 100 mg) for children weighing less than 45 kg. If weighing more than 45 kg, the adult dose should be used. The risk of dental staining is low in short course of therapy.
- Chloramphenicol 50 mg/kg per day in 4 divided doses (maximum of 4 g) is the preferred antibiotic in pregnancy, and the only alternative to doxycycline.[23] However, it is not readily available, and treatment with doxycycline should not be delayed if patient is severely ill.[23] In addition, only doxycycline should be given in the third trimester owing to potential of "gray baby" syndrome in the neonate with chloramphenicol exposure.

Therapy should be initiated within 5 days of onset of symptoms.[19]

Prevention

Prevention of tick bite is the same as recommended for Lyme disease. Currently, there is no vaccine available.

SUMMARY

Tickborne infections are common throughout much of the United States. The diagnosis can be challenging, because the presentation, history, and clinical examination findings can be mistaken for other illnesses, missed owing to negative initial testing or not considered in the differential diagnosis. Clinicians need to take a thorough history of patients presenting with fevers, rashes, joint pains, or other examination findings that may indicate tick exposure and subsequent infection. Patients may not recall a specific tick bite, but treatment should not be delayed in a symptomatic patient if clinical suspicion of tickborne infection is strong. In addition, for patients who do not respond to antibiotic therapy, coinfection with other tickborne infections should be considered, and appropriate testing and treatment initiated.

REFERENCES

1. Centers for Disease Control and Prevention. Lyme disease. Available at: http://www.cdc.gov/lyme. Accessed June 5, 2016.
2. Bratton R, Whiteside J, Hovan M, et al. Diagnosis and treatment of Lyme disease. Mayo Clin Proc 2008;83(5):566–71.
3. Shapiro E. Lyme disease. N Engl J Med 2014;370:1724–31.
4. Wormser G, Dattwyler R, Shapiro E, et al. The clinical assessment, treatment and prevention of Lyme disease, human granulocytic anaplasmosis, and babesiosis: clinical practice guidelines by the Infectious Diseases Society of America. Clin Infect Dis 2006;43(9):1089–134.
5. Evans J, Malawista S. Lyme disease. In: Schlossberg D, editor. Clinical infectious disease. New York: Cambridge University Press; 2008. p. 1127–34.
6. Stanek G, Wormser G, Gray J, et al. Lyme borreliosis. Lancet 2012;379(9814):461.
7. Sanchez E, Vannier E, Wormser G, et al. Diagnosis, treatment and prevention of Lyme disease, human granulocytic anaplasmosis and Babesiosis. JAMA 2016; 315(16):1767–77.
8. Logigian E, Kaplan R, Steere A. Chronic neurologic manifestations of Lyme disease. N Engl J Med 1990;323:1438–44.
9. Hu L. Clinical manifestations of Lyme disease in adults. In: Steere A, editor. UpToDate. Waltham (MA): UpToDate. Available at: www.uptodate.com. Accessed April 3, 2016.
10. Lelovas P, Dontas I, Bassiakou E, et al. Cardiac implications of Lyme disease, diagnosis and therapeutic approach. Int J Cardiol 2008;129(1):15–21.
11. Lantos P, Auwaerter P, Nelson C. Lyme disease serology. JAMA 2016;315(16): 1780–1.
12. Callister S, Jobe D, Stuparic-Stancic A, et al. Detection of IFN-gamma secretion by T cells collected before and after successful treatment of early Lyme disease. Clin Infect Dis 2016;62(10):1235–41.
13. Vannier E, Krause P. Human babesiosis. N Engl J Med 2012;366:2397–407.
14. Chen T, Krause P. Human babesiosis. In: Schlossberg D, editor. Clinical infectious disease. New York: Cambridge University Press; 2008. p. 1381–7.
15. Gelfand J, Vannier E. Clinical manifestations, diagnosis, treatment and prevention of Babesiosis. In: Daily J, editor. UpToDate. Waltham (MA): UpToDate. Available at: www.uptodate.com. Accessed June 15, 2016.
16. Dumler J, Madigan J, Pusterla N, et al. Ehrlichiosis in humans: epidemiology, clinical presentation, diagnosis and treatment. Clin Infect Dis 2007;45(1):S45–51.
17. Centers for Disease Control and Prevention. Anaplasma treatment and diagnosis. Available at: http://www.cdc.gov/anaplasmosis/symptoms. Accessed May 17, 2016.
18. Dhand A, Nadelman R, Aguero-Rosenfeld M, et al. Human Granulocytic Anaplasmosis during pregnancy: case series and literature review. Clin Infect Dis 2007; 45:589–93.

19. Centers for Disease Control and Prevention. Tickborne diseases of the United States. A reference manual for health care providers, 3rd edition. 2015. Available at: http://www.cdc.gov. Accessed June 20, 2016.
20. Sexton D, McClain M. Clinical manifestations and diagnosis of Rocky Mountain spotted fever. In: Calderwood S, Kaplan S, editors. UpToDate. Waltham (MA): UpToDate. Available at: www.uptodate.com. Accessed June 1, 2016.
21. Walker D. Rocky mountain spotted fever: a seasonal alert. Clin Infect Dis 1995;20: 1111–7.
22. Walker D, Raoult D. Rickettsia rickettsii and other spotted fever group rickettsiae (Rocky Mountain spotted fever and other spotted fevers). In: Mandell GL, Bennett JE, Dolin R, editors. Mandell, Douglas and Bennett's principles and practice of infectious diseases. 5th edition. Philadelphia: Churchill Livingstone; 2005. p. 2035–43.
23. Sexton D. Treatment of Rocky Mountain spotted fever. In: Calderwood S, editor. UpToDate. Waltham (MA): UpToDate. Available at: www.uptodate.com. Accessed June 20, 2016.

Orthopedic Infections

Jamie R. Silkey, PA-C, MPAS, MHA[a],*, Stephanie L. Ludtke, PA-C, MPAS[b],
Kartikey Acharya, MD, MPH[c]

KEYWORDS

- Septic arthritis • Infectious arthritis • Orthopedic infections • Osteomyelitis
- Bone infections • Native joint infections

KEY POINTS

- The incidence of orthopedic infections is increasing owing to several population health factors.
- Orthopedic infections can be difficult to diagnose and treat owing to the nonspecific presentation and long list of differential diagnoses.
- The diagnosis and treatment of orthopedic infections is a multidisciplinary collaboration between orthopedic surgery, radiology, and infectious disease specialists.
- Treatment includes antibiotic therapy based on isolated pathogens; however, empiric therapy is often indicated in some clinical situations.

Orthopedic infections can be a frustrating situation for patients and a challenging diagnosis for clinicians. Infections of the joint and bone are increasing as a result of the increased incidence of diabetes and vascular disorders, as well as orthopedic surgeries. Orthopedic infections come in several forms with varying presentations and pathophysiologies.

INFECTIOUS ARTHRITIS OF NATIVE JOINTS
Definition

Infectious arthritis is a term used to describe an infection of a joint, usually caused by a microorganism. Infectious arthritis should be at the forefront of the differential diagnosis in patients presenting with 1 or more acutely swollen, painful, erythematous, warm joints, and is a medical emergency. Infectious arthritis carries substantial

---

The authors have nothing to disclose.
[a] Division of Foot and Ankle Surgery, Department of Orthopaedic Surgery, Medical College of Wisconsin, 9200 West Wisconsin Avenue, Specialty Clinics, 5th Floor, Milwaukee, WI 53226, USA; [b] Division of Joint Reconstruction, Department of Orthopaedic Surgery, Medical College of Wisconsin, 9200 West Wisconsin Avenue, Suite, Specialty Clinics, 5th Floor, Milwaukee, WI 53226, USA; [c] Division of Infectious Diseases, Medical College of Wisconsin, 9200 West Wisconsin Avenue, Suite 5100, Milwaukee, WI 53226, USA
* Corresponding author.
E-mail address: jsilkey@mcw.edu

Physician Assist Clin 2 (2017) 261–276
http://dx.doi.org/10.1016/j.cpha.2016.12.008
2405-7991/17/© 2016 Elsevier Inc. All rights reserved.

morbidity and mortality, especially when treatment is delayed or inadequate.[1,2] If not diagnosed and treated promptly, nongonococcal bacterial arthritis can lead to irreversible joint destruction.[3]

Epidemiology

The incidence of infectious arthritis in the general population is estimated to be around 2 to 5 cases per 100,000 persons per year.[4] The risk is higher in patients with inflammatory joint diseases like rheumatoid arthritis and patients with prior joint surgeries.[5] Given the increasing prevalence of joint surgeries and hence the at-risk population, there has been an increase in the worldwide incidence of infectious arthritis.[6]

Classification

Infectious arthritis can be classified based on duration of symptoms, microbiology, and route of infection. Acute-onset infectious arthritis is often secondary to bacterial, viral, or certain fungal infections. Chronic infectious arthritis is usually secondary to non-*Candida* fungal infections, tuberculosis, or nontuberculous mycobacterial infections. Pyogenic or bacterial infectious arthritis commonly occurs after hematogenous dissemination from endocarditis or bacteremia secondary to known or occult infective focus. Infectious arthritis can also be secondary to direct inoculation of microorganisms into the joint space and can complicate surgical procedures, intraarticular injections, and penetrating trauma or bite wounds. Finally, infectious arthritis can result from contiguous deep spread as a complication of skin and soft tissue infections.[7]

Risk Factors

The following risk factors increase the likelihood of developing infectious arthritis[1–3,5,8]:

- Age greater than 80 years,
- Diabetes mellitus,
- Rheumatoid arthritis,
- Osteoarthritis/degenerative joint disease,
- Prior intraarticular corticosteroid injections,
- Presence of prosthetic joint,
- Alcoholism,
- Intravenous (IV) drug use, and
- Skin disease/infections.

The most common predisposing conditions in the development of infectious arthritis are degenerative joint disease, rheumatoid arthritis, and corticosteroid therapy.[3] Patients with rheumatoid arthritis have an approximately 10-fold higher incidence of infectious arthritis than the general population.[3,6,9] Specific factors that put this patient population at increased risk include use of immunosuppressive therapy, glucocorticoids, and disease-modifying antirheumatic drugs.[6,9]

Pathophysiology

The pathophysiology of infectious arthritis depends on the route of infection and the microorganism involved. Several host factors, including local (joint-related factors including prior surgery) and systemic (age, comorbidities, and immune deficiencies), are at play in the pathogenesis of these infections. Factors unique to each microorganism, such as synovial tissue tropism and toxin production lead to synovial damage. Much of our understanding regarding the pathogenesis of nongonococcal infectious arthritis comes from animal models of these infections with *Staphylococcus aureus*.[10]

After hematogenous seeding or direct inoculation, the first step in pathogenesis involves the adherence of microorganisms to synovial tissue. Prominent vascularity along with a lack of protective basement membrane makes the synovium vulnerable to hematogenous seeding of microorganisms. In addition, certain organisms like S aureus also have tropism to synovial tissue. S aureus has surface receptors, such as fibronectin-binding protein and microbial surface components recognizing adhesive matrix molecules that facilitate adherence to extracellular matrix of joints.[3] Preexisting joint disease or injury leads to increased production and subsequent exposure of these matrix proteins to microorganisms.

After attachment, microorganisms invade the joint capsule and lead to an inflammatory response. The degree of host inflammatory response is the determining factor in joint damage and destruction that ensues. Uninterrupted, this can lead to intraarticular cartilage destruction, synovial ischemia, subsequent synovial necrosis, and eventual damage to the bone.[11]

In gonococcal arthritis, infection of the joint occurs after occult bacteremia that ensues after a mucosal site infection. It is usually seen as a part of the spectrum of disseminated gonococcal infections, and occurs in 1% to 3% of patients with asymptomatic mucosal site infection. As with nongonococcal infectious arthritis, apart from several organism-specific factors, some unique host factors play a role in pathogenesis of these infections. Disseminated gonococcal arthritis is particularly seen in hosts with immunodeficiency, especially related to terminal complement complex C5-8.[12]

Clinical Manifestations

A patient with suspected infectious arthritis classically presents with an acutely swollen, painful joint.[1] Patients usually describe a 1- to 2-week history of a red, painful joint.[2,9] Joint pain and joint swelling are the most common symptoms of infectious arthritis; fever is present in up to 60% of patients.[1] Sweats and rigors are seen less commonly in infectious arthritis.[1]

The most commonly affected joints in infectious arthritis are the knee and the hip, followed by the shoulder and ankle.[2,3] Nongonococcal arthritis is monoarticular in 80% to 90% of cases.[3] Involvement of the sternoclavicular, costochondral, and sacroiliac joints are more common in IV drug users.[3] Infectious arthritis of atypical joints tends to be proceeded by penetrating trauma, including bites and local corticosteroid therapy.[3]

Differential Diagnoses

Various other conditions presenting with similar symptoms of infectious arthritis should be considered in the evaluation of a swollen, painful, stiff joint. A list of conditions that should be included in the differential diagnosis of infectious arthritis is included in Box 1.

Diagnostic options

Patients who present with a history and examination concerning for infectious arthritis require further evaluation with diagnostic testing. It is widely accepted that the gold standard test for the diagnosis of infectious arthritis is arthrocentesis and joint fluid analysis.[1–3,5,6,8,9,13] The diagnosis of infectious arthritis relies on the isolation of the pathogen(s) from aspirated joint fluid.[3] Attention should be taken during arthrocentesis to avoid puncturing the joint through an area of skin that seems to be infected or erythematous, so as to avoid introducing contaminants into the joint or false-positive findings.[5]

The 2 tests most indicative of infectious arthritis are synovial fluid white blood cell count and percentage of polymorphonuclear cells. White blood cell counts of greater

---

Box 1
Differential diagnosis of infectious arthritis

Soft tissue infection

Rheumatoid arthritis

Gout

Pseudogout

Reactive arthritis

Systemic lupus erythematosus

Lyme arthritis

Sickle cell disease

Metastatic carcinoma

Pigmented villonodular synovitis

Hemarthrosis

Osteoarthritis

Intraarticular injury

Endocarditis

Charcot neuroarthropathy

Data from Margaretten ME, Kohlwes J, Moore D, et al. Does this adult patient have septic arthritis? JAMA 2007;297(13):1478–88; and Shirtliff ME, Mader JT. Acute septic arthritis. Clin Microbiol Rev 2002;15(4):527–44.

---

than 50,000/μL and a polymorphonuclear cell count of at least 90% are highly diagnostic of infectious arthritis.[1,3,8]

Joint fluid should also be sent for aerobic, anaerobic, mycobacterial, and fungal cultures. Gram stain may support the diagnosis of infectious arthritis, but is only effective 50% of the time, whereas cultures are positive in nongonococcal arthritis about 90% of the time. A recent study suggested that synovial fluid should be allowed an incubation time of at least 4 days before considering them to be negative.[13] Antibiotic sensitivities should be determined to help guide appropriate pharmacologic treatment.[3]

Synovial fluid glucose, protein, and lactate dehydrogenase levels have not been found to be directly diagnostic of infectious arthritis, and their validity in the evaluation of infectious arthritis has been questioned.[1,8] Although low joint fluid glucose levels and high lactate levels are nonspecific, they should create suspicion for infectious arthritis.[3,5,9]

Synovial fluid should also be examined for crystals to rule out crystalline joint disease such as gout and pseudogout.[2,3,9] Compensated polarizing light microscopy will show negatively birefringent uric acid crystals and positively birefringent calcium pyrophosphate dehydrate crystals in cases of gout and pseudogout, respectively. It is important, however, to note that simultaneous bacterial infection and crystalline disease have been reported.[3]

Most patients with infectious arthritis will also have elevated C-reactive protein levels and erythrocyte sedimentation rates.[2,3] Peripheral blood leukocyte counts are often within normal limits, but may be increased in children.[3]

Radiography has not been found to be useful in the acute stage of infectious arthritis.[5] However, various radiographic studies may be performed to help to identify any current or potential late sequelae. Plain radiographs may help to identify underlying joint destruction or preexisting disease. MRI can help in the evaluation of concurrent osteomyelitis, which may indicate the need for more advanced treatment.[5] MRI may also be useful in identifying the location of purulent material in the surrounding soft tissues near the primary joint infection.[2]

TREATMENT
Medical Treatment

The management of pyogenic infectious arthritis requires prompt drainage in addition to targeted antimicrobial therapy (Table 1). Soon after synovial fluid cultures have been obtained, antimicrobial therapy should be initiated. Based on synovial fluid

Table 1
Recommended empiric antimicrobial regimens for infectious arthritis

Gram Stain	Preferred antibiotic[a]	Additional Comments
Gram-positive cocci	IV vancomycin 15–20 mg/kg per dose every 8–12 h[1]	If allergic to vancomycin, consider IV daptomycin therapy and also consider infectious disease consultation. Typical duration of therapy is at least 4 wk for *S aureus* infection.
Gram-negative cocci	IV ceftriaxone 1 g every 24 h	For penicillin-allergic patients, possible empiric options include IV/PO ciprofloxacin or PO azithromycin. Typical duration of therapy for gonococcal arthritis is 1 wk.
Gram-negative bacilli	IV cefepime 2 g every 8 h or IV ceftazidime 2 g every 8 h	For penicillin-allergic patients,[2] possible options include IV aztreonam or IV meropenem or IV/PO fluoroquinolones (levofloxacin/ciprofloxacin).[3] If concern for gram-negative resistance, including ESBL-producing organisms is high, consider parenteral carbapenem therapy (meropenem or imipenem if concerned for *Pseudomonas* infection, ertapenem if concern for *Pseudomonas* infection is low).
Gram-stain negative	IV vancomycin 15–20 mg/kg per dose every 8–12 h[1] plus IV cefepime or IV ceftazidime	

Therapeutic drug monitoring should always be done for patients on IV vancomycin therapy with targeted serum trough of 15 to 20 mg/L.

For patients with life-threatening allergy and/or known severe immunoglobulin E-mediated reaction to beta-lactam, IV aztreonam is the preferred agent for gram-negative coverage. Although cross-reactivity is low, caution is advised in the use of carbapenem therapy (eg, IV meropenem) in patients with history of penicillin or cephalosporin allergy.[40,41]

Caution is advised when fluoroquinolone therapy is used along with other agents that prolong QT interval. Consider doing an electrocardiogram at baseline in these patients.

Azithromycin is a possible alternative for patients with suspected gonococcal arthritis and history of penicillin allergy.[7]

Abbreviations: ESBL, extended spectrum beta lactamase; IV, intravenous(ly); PO, orally.
[a] All dosages for antimicrobials listed are for individuals with normal renal function.

Adapted from Ohl CA, Forster D. Infectious Arthritis of Native Joints. In: Bennett JE, Dolin R, Blaser MJ, editors. Mandell, Douglas and Bennett's principles and practice of infectious diseases. 8th edition. Philadelphia: Elsevier Saunders; 2015. p. 1302–17; with permission.

culture and susceptibility testing results, empiric antimicrobial therapy may be tailored as needed.

Empiric therapy should be initiated based on knowledge of epidemiologic factors along with synovial fluid gram stain data. Even in patients with negative gram stain, empiric antimicrobial therapy should be started if clinical concern of Infectious arthritis is high.

Given the high prevalence of staphylococcal infections, including community-acquired methicillin-resistant S aureus, empiric IV vancomycin should be initiated in cases where the synovial fluid gram stain shows gram positive cocci or if the synovial fluid gram stain is negative. Parenteral antipseudomonal cephalosporins (eg, cefepime, ceftazidime) should be started if synovial fluid gram stain shows gram negative bacilli. If the prevalence of gram-negative resistance is high, carbapenem therapy (imipenem or meropenem if Pseudomonas infection suspected) should be considered.

The duration of therapy depends on individual microorganisms, certain host factors, and clinical response. Methicillin-resistant S aureus and gram-negative bacilli infections need 4 to 6 weeks of antimicrobial therapy after adequate surgical drainage, whereas for disseminated gonococcal arthritis, 1 week of antimicrobial therapy with a parenteral third-generation cephalosporin (eg, ceftriaxone) is generally sufficient.[2,5]

Parenteral therapy is preferred for antimicrobial therapy of infectious arthritis. However, certain drugs like linezolid and fluoroquinolones (eg, levofloxacin, ciprofloxacin) have excellent oral bioavailability and could be used to shorten the parenteral antimicrobial course if the organism is susceptible to these agents. Fluoroquinolones should never be used alone in treatment of staphylococcal joint infections owing to rapid emergence of resistance while on treatment. With therapy lasting longer than 2 weeks, linezolid use can be associated with reversible myelosuppression and peripheral neuropathy. Rare cases of optic neuropathy have been also been described with prolonged use of linezolid. For methicillin-resistant S aureus infectious arthritis, IV vancomycin is the preferred drug. However, if the minimum inhibitory concentration of vancomycin is greater than or equal to 1 mg/L, the chances of failure with vancomycin are high. In certain cases with poor response, alternate antimicrobials like daptomycin should be considered.[2,7]

Nonbacterial infectious arthritis can be secondary to viral infection, fungal infection, and mycobacterial infections. An infectious disease consultation should be obtained when there is a suspected or proven case of acute or chronic arthritis secondary to these nonbacterial organisms.

Surgical Treatment Options

In addition to antimicrobial therapy, drainage of the joint is often indicated in the treatment of infectious arthritis to help remove purulent material.[2,3,6,8,9] Various options for the method of drainage exist, but evidence for the most effective procedure is limited,[2] and there is no definitive evidence to recommend 1 method over the other.[8] Procedures include needle aspiration, arthroscopy, and arthrotomy.[3]

Initially, needle aspiration (arthrocentesis) is the preferred treatment option and is the procedure used to help confirm the diagnosis of infectious arthritis.[3,9] Recurrent effusions occurring in the first 7 days may be amenable to repeated needle aspiration; however, a persistent effusion past 7 days is an indication that a more invasive surgical procedure may be necessary.[3]

Arthroscopy has been used increasingly in the treatment of infectious arthritis of the knee and hip. Arthroscopy is less invasive than an arthrotomy and provides better visualization and irrigation than needle aspiration alone.[3] Arthroscopy is also associated with a quicker recovery and less morbidity.[8]

Arthrotomy is the procedure of choice when urgent decompression of the joint is needed owing to neuropathy or vascular compromise.[3] Other indications for arthrotomy include failure of other less invasive methods, advanced joint destruction by preexisting disease, and concurrent osteomyelitis requiring debridement.[3]

Summary

Infectious arthritis is an urgent condition requiring timely evaluation and treatment. Patients with signs and symptoms suspicious for infectious arthritis should undergo arthrocentesis for further evaluation and confirmation of the diagnosis. Identification of the offending pathogen is essential in determining the appropriate antimicrobial treatment regimen. Early treatment of infectious arthritis, both pharmacologic and procedural, is critical in the prevention of chronic infections or other long-term sequelae, including rapid joint degeneration.

OSTEOMYELITIS
Background

With descriptions dating back to the Hippocrates era (460–370 BC), osteomyelitis is one of the oldest diseases on record. The process was initially described as "abscessus in medulla," "necrosis," or "a boil of the bone marrow" until Nelaton coined the term *osteomyelitis* in 1844.[14] Osteomyelitis refers to the osseous inflammatory destruction and necrosis related to an infection localized to the bone.[15–18] Although bone is typically resistant to bacterial colonization, circumstances in which the soft tissue or bony integrity is disrupted, such as trauma, surgery, the presence of foreign bodies, placement of prostheses, or ulcers, may lead to the onset of a bone infection.

Until the 1940s, the management of acute osteomyelitis entailed large surgical excisions of all necrotic and infected bone with wounds packed and left to heal by secondary means.[14] During this time, mortality rates remained high (about 33%) owing to sepsis. With the introduction of penicillin in 1940, the treatment and prognosis of osteomyelitis shifted from containment to cure as complications such as sequestration, sinus formation, and sepsis became less common. In today's medicine, early and specific treatment through identification of causative microorganisms is essential to the outcomes of osteomyelitis treatment.[18]

Etiology

S aureus is the most common cause of osteomyelitis for the acute, chronic, hematogenous, and contiguous presentations, with the organism being identified in 30% to 60% of cases.[19–21] Other relevant organisms are based on the patient's age. *Group A Streptococcus*, *Streptococcus pneumoniae*, and *Kingella kingae* are common pathogens found in children, whereas *Staphylococcus epidermidis*, *Pseudomonas aeruginosa*, *Serratia marcescens*, *Escherichia coli*, and *Enterococcus spp*, are more commonly isolated in adults.[21,22] Some studies have reported methicillin-resistant *S aureus* accounting for as many as one-third of all staphylococcal isolates.[21] Fungal agents have also been reported, including *Candida* and *Aspergillus*; however, these are uncommon and typically present in the immunocompromised population.[21,22]

Risk Factors

Risk factors for osteomyelitis include diabetes mellitus, peripheral neuropathy, peripheral vascular disease, kidney disease, immunosuppression, and a history of open fracture or orthopedic surgery with hardware implantation.[23] Diabetic foot ulcers are among the most common causes of osteomyelitis, with 20% to 25% of patients with diabetic foot ulcers developing a bone infection.[22] Diabetes and peripheral vascular disease work synergistically to increase significantly the risk of osteomyelitis given the poor healing potential.[24] A major risk factor for vertebral osteomyelitis in adults is bacteremia secondary to injection drug use.[20]

Epidemiology

The incidence of osteomyelitis after an open injury is as high as 27% and is linked directly to the length of time from injury to surgery.[21] The standardization of preoperative preparations including antimicrobial shower, shaving, and skin preparation; the use of surgical rooms with laminar air flow; and prophylactic antibiotics have decreased the infection rate after orthopedic prosthetic surgery to 0.5% to 2.0% depending on the type of joint replacement.[16]

The incidence of osteomyelitis is higher in developing countries.[25] In the United States, the incidence is 21.8 cases per 1000 persons per year.[22] A recent study noted that the incidence of osteomyelitis remained relatively stable among children and young adults from 1969 to 2009; however, cases among older adults tripled in the same time period, likely driven by the increased prevalence of risk factors in that population, such as diabetes.[20]

Posttraumatic osteomyelitis accounts for approximately 47% of cases of osteomyelitis owing to high-energy open injuries and the use of orthopedic hardware. Other major causes of osteomyelitis include vascular insufficiency and neuropathic ulcers commonly seen in persons with diabetes (34%), and hematogenous seeding from bacteremia (19%).[26,27] Calcaneal osteomyelitis has been reported in 1.8% to 6.4% of patients after foot puncture wounds.[28]

Classification

There are several schemes for classification of osteomyelitis: the Cierny and Mader classification is helpful in staging osteomyelitis to help formulate treatment and prognosis for the infection. This classification includes information on extent of bone involvement along with local and systemic host factors that affect treatment.[29] Lew and Waldvogel's classification focuses more on the etiology of osteomyelitis: hematogenous versus contiguous (exogenous).[15] Hematogenous osteomyelitis is an infection that spreads to the bone from the bloodstream. Contiguous osteomyelitis implies a bone infection that was introduced from an external source, such as orthopedic hardware or infected soft tissue. Along with the mechanism of infection, this classification focuses on duration of illness and presence of peripheral vascular disease.[15]

From a management perspective, a combination of both staging schemes is important and helps to differentiate osteomyelitis into 3 groups: (a) osteomyelitis secondary to contiguous spread from open wound after trauma or surgery, (b) osteomyelitis secondary to vascular insufficiency, especially in patients with diabetes where bone infection follows necrotizing or nonnecrotizing soft tissue infection of foot, and (c) hematogenous osteomyelitis seen in patients with overt or occult bacteremia. The latter group could present with acute onset vertebral osteomyelitis or long bone osteomyelitis.[15]

Pathophysiology

The pathophysiology of osteomyelitis differs based on the location of the bone infection. It is important to realize that normal bone is resistant to infection. However, once infected, bone infections can tend to lead to ischemic necrosis of bone. Necrotic bone is the hallmark of chronic osteomyelitis.[16] After infection, pus spreads into the vascular channels, increases the intraosseous pressure, and impairs blood flow. What ensues is ischemic necrosis of the affected bone and results in formation of sequestra, which are fragments of devascularized bone tissue.[16]

Osteomyelitis of the foot is often seen in patients with diabetes, peripheral arterial insufficiency, or peripheral neuropathy and a history of foot surgery or a pressure ulcer.[24] These infections are common in patients with poorly controlled diabetes mellitus who typically have a constellation of risk factors in form of vasculopathy, neuropathy, and relative immune deficiency. These groups of bone infections are acquired almost exclusively by the exogenous or contiguous route.

Vertebral osteomyelitis and osteomyelitis of the long bones is often a consequence of hematogenous seeding after an episode of bacteremia. Vertebral osteomyelitis is often referred to as spinal osteomyelitis or disk space infection and starts with bacterial seeding of vertebral endplates that spreads into the vertebral disk. Occasionally, vertebral osteomyelitis is also seen complicating spinal surgery or trauma when the source of infection is exogenous.[30] Hematogenous infection in long bones typically occurs in children and older adults[17] with more than 50% of cases in children less than 5 years of age.[21] Parenteral antibiotic therapy is preferred, especially for the treatment of hematogenous osteomyelitis. Inadequate treatment can lead frequently to relapses in these cases, sometimes even 80 years after initial infection.[31]

Clinical Manifestations

Acute osteomyelitis may present with a gradual onset of erythema, warmth, and edema over the affected bone and is associated more commonly with constitutional symptoms in children than adults. Subacute osteomyelitis generally presents with onset of mild pain over several weeks, minimal fever, and few constitutional symptoms. Chronic osteomyelitis may present with pain, erythema, or swelling, and an associated wound, but frequently lacks constitutional symptoms.[24]

Hematogenous osteomyelitis presents differently than contiguous osteomyelitis. Children with hematogenous osteomyelitis tend to present more acutely, typically within 2 weeks of the gradual onset of systemic symptoms including fever, malaise, and irritability.[24] Pain in the affected limb and adjacent joint with decreased motion, edema, and erythema over the involved area may be noted on physical examination. Adults with hematogenous osteomyelitis may present with a primary complaint of back pain. Hematogenous osteomyelitis typically involves the vertebrae, but can present in the long bones, pelvis, or clavicle.[24]

Contiguous osteomyelitis can be nonspecific in presentation and difficult to recognize. Patients typically have an associated wound and may present with chronic pain, persistent sinus tract or wound drainage, poor wound healing, malaise, or occasional fever; however, constitutional symptoms, such as fever, chills, nausea, and vomiting, are not common on presentation. The classic signs of inflammation, including local pain, swelling, or redness, may also occur and normally disappear within 5 to 7 days.[24] Underlying osteomyelitis should be suspected in patients with exposed bone, persistent sinus tract, tissue necrosis overlying bone, chronic wound overlying surgical hardware, and chronic wound overlying fracture.[21]

The suspicion of osteomyelitis should be raised in diabetic patients with soft tissue inflammation or skin ulcerations over bony prominences.[15] Diabetic patients may present without fever and with few signs of inflammation, and require careful assessment of the vascular supply to the affected limb and any concomitant neuropathy. Deep or extensive ulcers that fail to heal after several weeks of appropriate ulcer care, should raise suspicion for chronic osteomyelitis.[32] In the presence of a chronic wound, probe to the bone or exposed bone may be sufficient for the diagnosis of osteomyelitis. Some studies report that the probe-to-bone test has a 66% sensitivity, 85%

specificity, 89% positive predictive value, and 56% negative predictive value in diagnosing osteomyelitis.[32] In the diabetic population, however, this test may have a lower positive predictive value and other noninvasive imaging may be necessary to confirm the diagnosis.[33] The absence of a positive probe-to-bone test may be sufficient to exclude the diagnosis.[33]

Differential Diagnosis

The differential diagnosis of osteomyelitis includes:[34]

- Soft tissue infection (cellulitis),
- Charcot neuroarthropathy,
- Osteonecrosis (avascular necrosis of bone),
- Inflammatory arthritis (gout, pseudogout, psoriasis, rheumatoid arthritis),
- Fracture,
- Bursitis, and
- Malignancy.

If osteomyelitis is suspected based on clinical history and physical findings, diagnostic studies including imaging, laboratory tests, and cultures are indicated.

Diagnostic Options

The diagnosis of osteomyelitis can be difficult and requires a multidisciplinary approach including imaging, laboratory medicine, and pathology[21] (Table 2).

Conventional radiographs are the initial imaging study of choice at presentation and follow-up of acute osteomyelitis, which may show soft tissue swelling, narrowing or widening of joint spaces, bone destruction, sclerosis, and periosteal reaction (Fig. 1) approximately 10 to 21 days after the onset of infection.[16] At least 50% to 75% of the bone matrix must be destroyed for lytic changes to be seen on radiographs; thus, negative radiographic studies do not exclude the diagnosis of acute osteomyelitis.[25]

Ultrasonography may be helpful in the early diagnosis of osteomyelitis before radiographic changes are visible.[22] Ultrasonic evidence of acute osteomyelitis includes deep soft tissue swelling, periosteal thickening and elevation, and subperiosteal fluid collection.

Given the excellent resolution, both computed tomography and MRI can reveal the destruction of medulla, periosteal reaction, cortical destruction, articular damage, and soft tissue involvement, despite normal conventional radiographs.[15] Computed tomography is extremely useful for guiding needle biopsy or identification of sequestra. MRI is more useful than computed tomography for soft tissue involvement and its sensitivity for bone marrow edema can be useful in the detection of an early infection. However, MRI may not be as helpful in assessing the response to therapy, given that bone marrow edema can persist for many months despite microbiological cure. MRI bone marrow edema findings are nonspecific with similar results originating from tumors, fractures, and other inflammatory process such as Charcot neuroarthropathy, leading to specificity as low as 60%.[15,21]

Nuclear medicine imaging can offer the greatest specificity and sensitivity; however, access to these tests may be limited by location and cost.[21] The use of a routine bone scintigraphy may frequently yield a false-positive in the presence of Charcot neuroarthropathy, gout, trauma, and surgery. However, combining radiopharmaceutical tagged white blood cell scans (indium-111) with bone scintigraphy (technetium-99m) can detect acute osteomyelitis with 100% sensitivity and 81% specificity

Table 2
Diagnostic imaging studies for osteomyelitis[21,35]

Imaging Modality	Sensitivity (%)	Specificity (%)	Comments
Plain radiographs (anterior-posterior, lateral, oblique)	14–54	68–70	Useful to rule out other pathology
MRI	78–90	60–90	Useful to distinguish between soft tissue and bone infection. Increased sensitivity may lead to false positives. Less useful in cases with retained hardware owing to artifact.
Computed tomography	67	50	Generally not useful for osteomyelitis evaluation unless to guide biopsy
Technetium-99 bone scintigraphy (bone scan)	82	25	Specificity is improved when bone scan and indium scan are done in conjunction
Leukocyte scintigraphy (Indium 111)	61–84	60–84	
Technetium-99 bone scintigraphy (bone scan) + leukocyte scintigraphy (Indium 111)	100	84	A 2-d test. Extremely useful in differentiating osteomyelitis from other destructive bony process such as Charcot neuroarthropathy. Results may be compromised with peripheral arterial disease.
PET	96	91	Expensive, limited availability

Data from Hatzenbuehler J, Pulling T. Diagnosis and management of osteomyelitis. Am Fam Physician 2011;84(9):1027–33; and Eisenberg, B, Wrege SS, Altman MI, et al. Bone scan: indium-WBC correlation in the diagnosis of osteomyelitis of the foot. J Foot Surg 1989;28(6):532–36

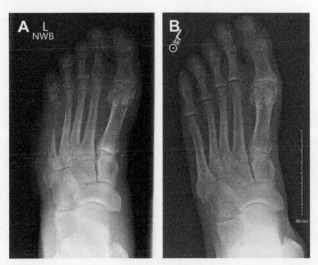

Fig. 1. Radiographic evidence of osteomyelitis. Fifth metatarsal osteomyelitis (*A*) compared with a normal foot radiograph (*B*). (*Courtesy of* R. Marks, MD, Milwaukee, WI.)

(Fig. 2).[35] PET has the greatest sensitivity and a specificity of greater than 90%, but is expensive and not as widely available.[21]

Laboratory data

White blood cell counts are not a reliable indicator of osteomyelitis because leukocytes rarely exceed 15,000/μL acutely, and are usually normal in chronic osteomyelitis.[15,24,25] Although the erythrocyte sedimentation rate is high in most cases of osteomyelitis, C-reactive protein is a more reliable test when assessing the presence of infection and response to treatment because its concentration can change more rapidly.[15] C-reactive protein and erythrocyte sedimentation rate levels may be elevated in other scenarios unrelated to osteomyelitis, but a persistently normal erythrocyte sedimentation rate and C-reactive protein virtually rules out the diagnosis of osteomyelitis.[21] Serum calcium, phosphate, and alkaline phosphatase levels are normal in osteomyelitis in contrast with metastatic or metabolic bone disease.[15]

Cultures

In cases with high clinical suspicion for osteomyelitis and evidence of an infection on imaging modalities, bone biopsy with histopathologic examination and culture is the gold standard to confirm the diagnosis and to guide antimicrobial therapy. Bone biopsy leads to a definitive diagnosis by isolating pathogens directly from the bone lesion.[24] Bone biopsies should be performed through uninvolved tissue and ideally either before the initiation of antibiotics or more than 48 hours after discontinuation.

A bone biopsy may not be indicated for patients with radiologic studies consistent with osteomyelitis and positive blood cultures; however, blood cultures are positive in only 50% of cases of osteomyelitis.[24] Open biopsy is preferable over needle biopsy. In circumstances where surgical debridement is required, bone samples should be obtained at the time of surgical debridement.[36] Percutaneous bone biopsies should be performed through intact uninvolved tissues with fluoroscopic or computed tomography guidance to obtain accurate culture results.[37]

Cultures of superficial wounds and sinus tracts do not correlate reliably with pathogens in the underlying bone.[38] Only 44% of sinus tract cultures contained the pathogen isolated from a deep surgical specimen.[38] Although sinus tract cultures do not

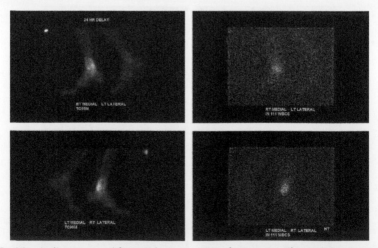

Fig. 2. Positive indium scan with correlating positive bone scan. The positive tagged white blood cell scans (indium-111) (*Right*) of the fibula with correlating inflammation on the bone scintigraphy (technetium-99m) (*Left*). (*Courtesy of* R. Marks, MD, Milwaukee, WI.)

predict the presence of gram-negative organisms, they are helpful in confirming *S aureus* infection.

Treatment

The treatment of osteomyelitis consists of the implementation of appropriate antibiotic therapy and, frequently, surgical intervention for removal of infected and necrotic tissue. The curative process includes input from a multidisciplinary team, including experts in infectious diseases, radiology, orthopedic surgery, and plastic surgery.

Cultures can determine antibiotic therapy; however, in the absence of culture data, empiric, broad-spectrum antibiotics should be administered (Table 3). Delaying

Table 3
Treatment principles and antimicrobial regimens for osteomyelitis

Clinical Setting	Treatment[a]	Additional Comments
Osteomyelitis of foot secondary to direct injury to bone from trauma or surgery	Suggested antimicrobial regimen: IV vancomycin 15–20 mg/kg per dose every 8–12 h[1] plus IV cefepime 2 g every 8–12 h	Antimicrobial therapy should follow wound irrigation and debridement. Infections are often polymicrobial in nature: empiric coverage against staphylococci and aerobic gram-negative bacilli is warranted. These infections are generally chronic in nature.
Osteomyelitis of extremities in patients with peripheral vascular disease (including diabetic foot infections); secondary to contiguous spread from adjacent soft tissue infection	Suggested antimicrobial regimen: IV vancomycin 15–20 mg/kg per dose every 8–12 h[1] plus IV piperacillin-tazobactam 4.5 g every 6 h	Emergent surgical debridement and removal of necrotic bone is needed in several cases. Infections are polymicrobial in nature: empiric coverage against methicillin-resistant *S aureus*, streptococci, aerobic gram-negative bacilli and anaerobic organisms is needed. Revascularization options should be considered in patients with peripheral vascular disease.
Hematogenous osteomyelitis of long bones or vertebral osteomyelitis	Suggested antimicrobial regimens would be targeting the organism involved in bloodstream infection: Methicillin-sensitive *S aureus* – consider nafcillin sodium 2 g IV every 4 h Methicillin-resistant *S aureus* – Consider IV vancomycin 15–20 mg/kg per dose every 8–12 h[1] *Pseudomonas aeruginosa* – consider IV cefepime 2 g IV every 8 h	These infections are usually monomicrobial in nature. These infections are generally acute in nature and blood cultures are often positive. Additional workup may be needed for bacteremia. Antimicrobial therapy alone may be adequate in several of these cases; unless there are complications and significant surrounding soft tissue infection.

Therapeutic drug monitoring should always be done for patients on IV vancomycin therapy with a targeted serum trough of 15 to 20 mg/L.

Abbreviation: IV, intravenous(ly).

[a] In all cases, try obtaining culture data before starting empiric antimicrobial regimen.

Adapted from Berbari EF, Steckelberg JM, Osmon DR. Osteomyelitis. In: Mandell, Douglas, and Bennett's principles and practice of infectious diseases, 8th edition, Bennett E, Dolin R, Blaser M. Philadelphia: Saunders; 2015. p. 1318–27; with permission.

antibiotic administration until cultures and sensitivities are obtained may be considered given the high rate of false-negative cultures after the institution of antibiotic therapy.[21]

The duration of antibiotic therapy depends on presentation and age. In children with hematogenous osteomyelitis, therapy may consist of 4 days of IV antibiotics followed by oral antibiotics for a total of 4 weeks of therapy.[21] Immunocompromised children may require 6 weeks of antibiotic therapy given the higher recurrence rate in this population. The optimal duration and delivery route for adults is unknown.[21] General recommendations for parenteral antibiotics range from 2 to 6 weeks with a transition to oral antibiotics for a total of 4 to 8 weeks of treatment; however, the reoccurrence rate for chronic osteomyelitis in adults is 30% at 12 months.

Surgical indications include antibiotic failure, infected surgical hardware, and chronic osteomyelitis with necrotic bone and soft tissue.[21] Chronic osteomyelitis generally cannot be eradicated without surgical treatment. The goal of surgery is to achieve a viable vascularized environment, eliminate necrotic bone and tissue, and remove hardware that microorganisms may adhere to.[16]

Adequate debridement of necrotic bone can leave a large void that must be managed to prevent recurrence and bone instability.[16] Bone defects treated with bone fillers with or without antibiotic beads have a high success rate of 86% to 92%.[22] Large resections may also require extensive soft tissue coverage by plastic surgery such as skin grafts, muscle and myocutaneous flaps, and free flaps.[39]

Summary

Although relatively uncommon, osteomyelitis should be considered in high-risk populations such as diabetics with ulcers over bony prominences or nonhealing wounds after orthopedic surgeries. Given the nonspecific presentation of osteomyelitis, there are several differential diagnoses to consider. Clinical correlation with laboratory tests and imaging studies are required to make the presumptive diagnosis of osteomyelitis; bone cultures may be necessary to confirm the diagnosis. A multidisciplinary team is necessary for the successful treatment of osteomyelitis.

SUMMARY

Orthopedic infections are a challenging diagnosis requiring a multidisciplinary treatment approach. Several laboratory and imaging studies are available to confirm the presence of infection and rule out differential diagnoses. Clinicians should have a high index of suspicion of orthopedic infections in high risk populations. Isolating the organism is key to formulating the appropriate antibiotic treatment regimen; however, some situations require empiric therapy.

REFERENCES

1. Margaretten ME, Kohlwes J, Moore D, et al. Does this adult patient have septic arthritis? JAMA 2007;297(13):1478–88.
2. Mathews CJ, Weston VC, Jones A, et al. Bacterial septic arthritis in adults. Lancet 2010;375:846–55.
3. Shirtliff ME, Mader JT. Acute septic arthritis. Clin Microbiol Rev 2002;15(4): 527–44.
4. Smith JW, Chalupa P, Shabaz HM. Infectious arthritis: clinical features, laboratory findings and treatment. Clin Microbiol Infect 2006;12:309–14.
5. Tarkowski A. Infectious arthritis. Best Pract Res Clin Rheumatol 2006;20(6): 1029–44.

6. Sharff KA, Richards EP, Townes JM. Clinical management of septic arthritis. Curr Rheumatol Rep 2013;15:332–40.
7. Ohl CA, Forster D. Infectious arthritis of native joints. In: Bennett JE, Dolin R, Blaser MJ, editors. Mandell, Douglas and Bennett's principles and Practice of infectious diseases. 8th edition. Philadelphia: Elsevier Saunders; 2015. p. 1302–17.
8. Horowitz DL, Katzap E, Horowitz S, et al. Approach to septic arthritis. Am Fam Physician 2011;84(6):653–60.
9. Garcia-Arias M, Balsa A, Mola EM. Septic arthritis. Best Pract Res Clin Rheumatol 2011;25:407–21.
10. Tarkowski A, Collins LV, Gjertsson I, et al. Model systems: modeling human staphylococcal arthritis and sepsis in the mouse. Trends Microbiol 2001;9:321–6.
11. Roy S, Bhawan J. Ultrastructure of articular cartilage in pyogenic arthritis. Arch Pathol 1975;99:44–7.
12. Britigan BE, Cohen MS, Sparling PF. Gonococcal infection: a model of molecular pathogenesis. N Engl J Med 1985;312:1683–94.
13. Balderia PG, Pomerantz S, Fischer R. Acute bacterial arthritis: how long should you wait for culture results? J Clin Rheumatol 2015;21(4):196–8.
14. Klenerman L. A history of osteomyelitis from the Journal of Bone and Joint Surgery: 1948 to 2006. J Bone Joint Surg Br 2007;89(5):667–70.
15. Lew DP, Waldvogel FA. Osteomyelitis. Lancet 2004;364:369–79.
16. Lew DP, Waldvogel FA. Osteomyelitis. N Engl J Med 1997;336:999–1007.
17. Berbari EF, Steckelberg JM, Osmon DR. Osteomyelitis. In: Bennett E, Dolin R, Blaser M, editors. Mandell, Douglas, and Bennett's principles and Practice of infectious diseases. 8th edition. Philadelphia: Saunders; 2015. p. 1318–27.
18. Concia E, Prandini N, Massari L, et al. Osteomyelitis: clinical update for practical guidelines. Nucl Med Commun 2006;8:645–60.
19. Tong SY, Davis JS, Eichenberger E, et al. Staphylococcus aureus infections: epidemiology, pathophysiology, clinical manifestations, and management. Clin Microbiol Rev 2015;28(3):603–61.
20. Kremers HM, Nwojo ME, Ransom JE, et al. Trends in the epidemiology of osteomyelitis: a population-based study, 1969 to 2009. J Bone Joint Surg Am 2015;97(10):837–45.
21. Hatzenbuehler J, Pulling T. Diagnosis and management of osteomyelitis. Am Fam Physician 2011;84(9):1027–33.
22. Maffulli N, Papalia R, Zampogna B, et al. The management of osteomyelitis in the adult. Surgeon 2016;14(6):345–60.
23. Walter G, Kemmerer M, Kappler C, et al. Treatment algorithms for chronic osteomyelitis. Dtsch Arztebl Int 2012;109(14):257–64.
24. Paluska SA. Osteomyelitis. Clin Fam Pract 2004;6(1):127–56.
25. Calhoun JH, Manring MM. Adult osteomyelitis. Infect Dis Clin North Am 2005;19(4):765–86.
26. Roesgen M, Hierholzer G, Ilax PM. Post-traumatic osteomyelitis. Pathophysiology and management. Arch Orthop Trauma Surg 1989;108(1):1–9.
27. Böhm E, Josten C. What's new in exogenous osteomyelitis? Pathol Res Pract 1992;188(1–2):254–8.
28. Laughlin RT, Reeve F, Wright DG, et al. Calcaneal osteomyelitis caused by nail puncture wounds. Foot Ankle Int 1997;18(9):575–7.
29. Mader JT, Shirtliff M, Calhoun JH. Staging and staging application in osteomyelitis. Clin Infect Dis 1997;25:1303–9.
30. Zimmerli W. Vertebral osteomyelitis. N Engl J Med 2010;362:1022–9.

31. Gallie WE. First recurrence of osteomyelitis eighty years after infection. J Bone Joint Surg Br 1951;33-B:110–1.
32. Grayson ML, Gibbons GW, Balogh K, et al. Probing to bone in infected pedal ulcers: a clinical sign of underlying osteomyelitis in diabetic patients. JAMA 1995; 273:721–3.
33. Lavery LA, Armstrong DG, Peters E, et al. Probe-to-bone test for diagnosing diabetic foot osteomyelitis. Diabetes Care 2007;30:270–4.
34. Lalani T. Overview of osteomyelitis in adults. In: UpToDate, Sexton DJ, editors. Waltham (MA): UpToDate; 2016.
35. Eisenberg B, Wrege SS, Altman MI, et al. Bone scan: indium-WBC correlation in the diagnosis of osteomyelitis of the foot. J Foot Surg 1989;28(6):532–6.
36. Gordon L, Chiu EJ. Treatment of infected non-unions and segmental defects of the tibia with staged microvascular muscle transplantation and bone-grafting. J Bone Joint Surg Am 1988;70(3):377–86.
37. Howard CB, Einhorn M, Dagan R, et al. Fine-needle bone biopsy to diagnose osteomyelitis. J Bone Joint Surg Br 1994;76(2):311–4.
38. Pearson RL, Miller GA. Accuracy of cultures of material from swabbing of the superficial aspect of the wound and needle biopsy in the preoperative assessment of osteomyelitis. J Bone Joint Surg Am 1991;73(5):745–9.
39. Weiland AJ, Moore JR, Daniel RK. The efficacy of free tissue transfer in the treatment of osteomyelitis. J Bone Joint Surg Am 1984;66(2):181–93.
40. Gruchalla RS, Pirmohamed M. Antibiotic allergy. N Engl J Med 2006;354:601–9.
41. Kula B, Djordjevic G, Robinson JL. A systematic review: can one prescribe carbapenems to patients with IgE-mediated allergy to penicillins or cephalosporins? Clin Infect Dis 2014;59:1113–22.

Managing Common Bite Wounds and Their Complications in the United States

Kyle Kalchbrenner, PA-C, MPAS*

KEYWORDS

- Bite wound infection • *Pasteurella* • *Eikenella* • Bite prophylaxis
- Amoxicillin/clavulanic acid • Dog bite • Cat bite • Human bite

KEY POINTS

- Bite wounds are quite common in the United States, and have a high propensity for polymicrobial infection.
- Wound cultures in this setting can help narrow antibiotics by ruling out potential resistant organisms, but broad coverage of common aerobes and anaerobes is still necessary.
- Dog, cat, and human bites all have a tendency to occur on the upper extremities where there is limited overlying protective clothing and greater possibility of tendon and joint involvement.
- Antibiotic prophylaxis in uncomplicated, noninfected-appearing bite wounds has mixed data, but is recommended in multiple situations such as an immunocompromised patient.
- The need for rabies prophylaxis from domestic dog or cat bites in the United States is typically low, but varies by region and this should be evaluated on a case-by-case basis with help of local health departments.

INTRODUCTION

A patient is admitted to your service for an infected right hand bite wound that he sustained while attempting to pet his neighbor's new dog. He cleaned the wound thoroughly at home following the injury and applied some topical antibiotics. The next day his hand became significantly more red, swollen, and painful in the region of trauma. He also developed difficulty extending his index finger. Preliminary radiograph shows soft tissue swelling without foreign body. He is afebrile but has a mild leukocytosis to 13.2.

Clinicians in every setting will come across the often-complicated bite-related infection, and it is imperative to know the steps necessary to provide exceptional care for

The author has nothing to disclose.
PA Specializing in Infectious Diseases
* 15540 Kemper Drive, Orland Park, IL 60462.
E-mail address: kkalch2@gmail.com

Physician Assist Clin 2 (2017) 277–286
http://dx.doi.org/10.1016/j.cpha.2016.12.009
2405-7991/17/© 2016 Elsevier Inc. All rights reserved.

your patient. Working within the realm of infectious disease in this setting requires important critical thinking ability, but once learned can be mastered quite easily.

Throughout the course of this article, the focus is primarily on infected bites inflicted by the most common 3 sources: dogs, cats, and humans. The microbiology of each of these sources is discussed in detail, with special attention to the clinical manifestations of a typical bite-related infection along with potential complications depending on the depth and location of the wound, as well as individual host factors. The need for further evaluation including laboratory tests and diagnostics, and the treatment of the wound with any potential complication also is examined. Furthermore, it also is important to recognize and understand potential need for rabies vaccination in this unique context.

EPIDEMIOLOGY

Bite wounds in the United States have a modestly high incidence, with 1 study reporting nearly 1% of all emergency room visits being due to mammalian bites on an annual basis.[1] The most frequent cause is secondary to dogs in 85% to 90% of cases in the United States,[2] followed by cats accounting for 2% to 50% of cases,[3] and lastly humans. It has been estimated that 50% of Americans will suffer a bite wound at some point in their life, and it is well known that many bites are frequently unreported, as many of these are minor and the victims frequently do not seek any type of medical attention. In those that are reported, it is more common for a patient to have an underlying infection, especially when the patient presents more than 8 hours after the inciting injury.[4,5]

Each type of bite does have specific epidemiologic properties, including the most common genders affected, as well as the most common region of trauma. Nearly 4.5 million people are bitten by dogs yearly,[3] with children making up the most frequently bitten group.[2] Overall, there are approximately 10 to 20 bite-related deaths per year, with most of them being due to dogs.[2] Dog bites in children are typically localized to the head and neck, whereas in adults the extremities are the most frequent sites affected.[2] Cat bites are seen in the highest number in female individuals and are also most commonly involving the extremities.[2] Human bites are more common among young men, which are also found on the hands and extremities. Interestingly, most of these are occlusion bites (bites in which both the top and bottom jaws come together to cause the injury), with closed-fist injuries (the notorious "fight bite") only accounting for 7.7% of them.[6]

MICROBIOLOGY

The microbiology underlying each of these sources of an infected bite wound is quite variable for multiple reasons. The most commonly found pathogens within each of these wounds often mimics those bacteria that inhabit the oral cavity of the biting organism. Less frequently, those bacteria that are colonizing the victim's skin or those present in the surrounding environment can be potential pathogens.[7] One very important unifying detail about any wound of this nature is to remember that it is frequently polymicrobial, involving gram-positive, gram-negative, and anaerobic isolates.

With regard to dog and cat bites, the most frequently isolated species of bacteria is *Pasteurella*. Cat bites are found to be linked higher with *Pasteurella multocida,* whereas *Pasteurella canis* is the most common among dog bites. Other common aerobes typically found include streptococci, staphylococci, *Moraxella*, and *Neisseria*. Anaerobically, *Fusobacterium, Bacteroides, Porphyromonas*, and *Prevotella* can be seen, but 1 study[8] found that anaerobes were more common isolates if an abscess was found. As might be predicted, this same study noticed that staphylococci and streptococci were more frequently isolated in nonpurulent wounds with associated lymphangitis. Interestingly, cat scratches also may be considered to have a similar microbiome as their bites,[9] which is potentially due to the frequency of paw licking in the feline grooming rituals. Other bacteria of clinical, but less common, significance include *Capnocytophaga canimorsus,* which can cause overwhelming sepsis in immunocompromised hosts,[5] as well as *Bartonella henselae,* which is the cause of "cat scratch fever."

Human bites are frequently found to carry *Streptococcus* and *Staphylococcus* species, most commonly *Streptococcus anginosus* and *Staphylococcus aureus.* One study reports that *S anginosus* can be found in approximately 52% of human bite wounds.[6] *Eikenella corrodens* is also a common pathogenic isolate from these wounds; in fact, it is uncommon for this isolate to occur in dog and cat bites, much like it is uncommon to see *Pasteurella* species in human bite wounds. Anaerobes of significance include *Fusobacterium nucleatum* and *Peptostreptococcus,* both of which are seen more frequently in occlusional bites.[10] A careful history always should be taken with any laceration concerning for infection, especially on the hands and upper extremities, because occasionally the patient will reactively place the wound in his or her mouth after the injury. This simple act can alter the microbiome of the wound and ultimately have an effect on the patient's response to therapy. In addition, paronychia in a patient who bites his or her nails or fingers ought to be considered in this class as well.[11]

Wound cultures in the setting of a bite wound infection can be quite helpful, but are typically used more to rule out potential resistant pathogens. For instance, as this article is being written I have a patient whom I am treating for tenosynovitis of the fifth digit of the hand due to a dog bite infection. Cultures had been obtained from the wound and are currently growing a coagulase-negative *Staphylococci.* Now in this setting, treating the culture alone would be improper management, as it is possible that there are other organisms present that did not grow well in aerobic and more often anaerobic cultures. At this point in time, narrowing the spectrum of antibiotics to remove coverage of methicillin-resistant *Staphylococcus aureus* (MRSA), while maintaining broad-spectrum coverage of other likely pathogens described previously, is an appropriate option.

IDENTIFYING AN INFECTED WOUND

Bite wounds from any source can be quite ghastly in appearance, with severe tissue damage and loss being possible. Noting signs of infection is paramount in these and other wounds. Clinically one might observe frank purulence in the wound bed, edema, or periwound erythema with indistinct margins and tenderness characteristic of cellulitis (Fig. 1). There also may be some associated lymphangitic streaking, especially on extremities. The wound and periwound regions should be palpated to assess for fluctuance and induration typical of developing abscess or phlegmon. Often, patients who do not need immediate medical care, such as those whose wounds could be cared for at home initially, will more often come in with these clinical signs. One might also begin to experience fevers/chills or have leukocytosis in laboratory data.

GENERAL MANAGEMENT OF A BITE WOUND

The physical examination following a bite wound should be well documented and if possible include a diagram of sustained injuries. Given advances in medical technology, some institutions also have begun documenting wounds such as these with

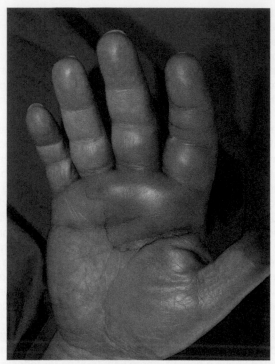

Fig. 1. Bite wound cellulitis. (*Courtesy of* Dr Rachel Rohde, Michigan Orthopaedic Institute, P.C. Royal Oak, MI.)

digital images that can be securely stored and can help the clinician monitor changes in the wound's status over time. On initial evaluation, it is important to document the type of animal, whether or not the bite was provoked, and when the incident occurred. Careful examination of the wound and its surrounding structures will give important clues regarding need for further evaluation.

The wound itself should be thoroughly cleaned with copious amounts of saline, and in the setting of puncture wounds it should be washed out with a jet of saline from a syringe. Any necrotic tissue should be debrided. Wounds are typically not primarily closed in this setting unless it appears clean and free of debris without evidence of infection on a region such as the face. General guidelines before primary closure typically include ensuring the wound does not appear infected, is less than 12 hours old, and is not located on the hand or foot. Importantly, cat and human bites ought to not be primarily closed unless they occur on the face and cosmesis is paramount.[12] On regions such as distal extremities, it is of utmost importance to elevate the site, as lack of this simple therapy can be a cause of treatment failure.[4]

THE ROLE OF ANTIBIOTIC PROPHYLAXIS IN SEEMINGLY UNCOMPLICATED BITE WOUNDS

It should be understood that there has been conflicting evidence to support the use of antibiotic prophylaxis in this setting. The Infectious Diseases Society of America (IDSA)[13] recommends the use in those who are immunocompromised or asplenic, in patients with advanced liver disease, when the affected region has significant chronic edema such as seen in a patient with mastectomy, in severe wounds, in injuries to the hand or face, and those wounds that have penetrated periosteum or a joint capsule. Those who are functionally asplenic, such as certain individuals with sickle cell anemia, also should be considered in this group.

Evaluation of an uncomplicated noninfected wound reveals tissue damage without evidence of significant edema, periwound erythema, lymphangitic streaking, fluctuant regions, or purulent drainage. The wound bed will be superficial, consist of clean tissue, and will be able to be completely evaluated without evidence of foreign bodies.

Dog bites have an overall lower infection rate than do cat and human bites, and it should be noted that all cat bites ought to be considered "high risk" and given prophylactic antibiotics. This would be due to the frequency of puncture wounds given the small size and sharp nature of feline dentition,[14,15] as well as the increased virulence of P multocida. If needed, prophylactic therapy should be continued for 3 to 5 days according to the IDSA.[13] Other sources recommend a 5-day to 7-day course of therapy.[14,15]

ANTIBIOTIC SELECTION

Antibiotic therapy for treatment of infected wounds, as well as antimicrobial selection for uncomplicated bite wound prophylaxis, should be directed toward the bacteria described previously. Prophylactic therapy will typically last for a 3-day to 7-day course as listed previously, whereas treatment of a truly infected wound without complication will range from 5 to 10 days, depending on response.[5,11] In the event that the patient has known MRSA colonization, this should be empirically covered as well. Initial MRSA therapy should be based on local resistance rates, and if available, previous cultures in the patient's history.

In the outpatient setting, an oral beta lactam/beta lactamase inhibitor, such as amoxicillin-clavulanic acid, is the only well-documented single drug choice for dog, cat, and human bites, as it will cover both Pasteurella and Eikenella species, as well as provide further gram-positive (including methicillin-sensitive S aureus and Streptococcus), gram-negative, and anaerobic coverage. It should be well understood that dicloxacillin, cephalexin, erythromycin, and clindamycin ought not to be used alone due to their inherent lack of activity against Pasteurella species.[14]

In the patient who is allergic to penicillin, or in those in whom MRSA is a consideration, various other regimens may be attempted but will typically require the use of 2 medications. Moxifloxacin, a fourth-generation fluoroquinolone, may be considered as monotherapy, as it provides broad coverage including most anaerobes found in these wounds, but activity against Bacteroides, Fusobacterium, and Prevotella species is variable.[16] Monotherapy of this nature is much less studied. Other antibiotics with activity against Pasteurella and Eikenella include doxycycline, trimethoprim-sulfamethoxazole (TMP-SMX), fluoroquinolones such as ciprofloxacin and levofloxacin, and in patients without type I hypersensitivity to penicillin, second-generation cephalosporins such as cefuroxime. Any of these can be paired with either metronidazole or clindamycin for anaerobic activity.

In the setting in which doxycycline is the antimicrobial agent chosen for Pasteurella/Eikenella coverage, it would be prudent to use clindamycin as the anaerobic drug of choice. This would be due to doxycycline having poor antistreptococcal activity. Similarly, if a fluoroquinolone is chosen, pairing it with clindamycin will also add further S aureus and streptococci coverage in light of emerging resistance patterns. Regimens including doxycycline, clindamycin, or TMP-SMX will provide MRSA coverage, but clindamycin susceptibilities will vary by local susceptibility rates. Remember to check your local resistance rates if using clindamycin, because some experts recommend avoiding its use if rates exceed 10% to 15% (Table 1).[17]

Table 1	
Antimicrobial options for prophylaxis and therapy	
Step 1: Choose an Antimicrobial Agent Directed Against *Pasteurella* or *Eikenella*	**Step 2: Choose an Antimicrobial Agent Directed Against Anaerobes**
Amoxicillin/clavulanic acid	Amoxicillin/clavulanic acid
Penicillin	Metronidazole
Cefuroxime doxycycline[a,b]	Clindamycin[a]
Trimethoprim-sulfamethoxazole[a]	
Ciprofloxacin, levofloxacin[b]	

Drug of choice: Will cover *Pasteurella*, *Eikenella*, methicillin-sensitive *Staphylococcus aureus*, streptococci, and also has appropriate anaerobic coverage.

[a] Will give empiric methicillin-resistant *S aureus* coverage.

[b] If using this drug, it would be prudent to pair it with clindamycin or amoxicillin/clavulanic acid to alleviate basic gaps in antimicrobial coverage.

In patients requiring hospitalization, intravenous options include ampicillin-sulbactam or piperacillin-tazobactam, a carbapenem such as ertapenem, a combination of ceftriaxone and metronidazole, or a combination of a fluoroquinolone, such as ciprofloxacin or levofloxacin and metronidazole. Vancomycin may be added to these regimens in the setting of known MRSA risk factors or history of carriage until culture results become available.[5,11]

When patients have pathology that requires prolonged intravenous therapy, it is important to also consider the frequency of dosing of the antibiotics to allow the patient to continue their activities of daily living, which will improve compliance and ensure optimal therapy. In this setting, so long as MRSA is not isolated, one single drug option is ertapenem, which is a carbapenem that is dosed once daily that has shown effective activity against common pathogens in both human and animal bite wounds.[18] Some of these complications that may require prolonged parenteral therapy are examined next.

COMPLICATIONS OF BITE WOUND INFECTIONS

It should be recognized that bite wounds in general have a significant rate of complication, and the clinician must always consider these possibilities. As described previously, bite wounds of all sources have a propensity for affecting the extremities in adults. Bites in these regions, especially the upper extremities, have risk of developing the complication of infectious arthritis or tenosynovitis. This relates to the large number of tendons and joints within the upper extremities, the fact that many of these structures are quite close to the surface of the skin, and the common lack of overlying protective clothing that is frequently apparent on the lower extremities, such as footwear.

In addition, the upper extremities are frequently used in combative or defensive situations, resulting in closed-fist injuries being located overlying the second, third, or fourth metacarpophalangeal (MCP) joints on the patient's dominant hand. It has been estimated that the MCP joint capsule is entered in 52% to 62% of this type of wound, and it is necessary to recognize that if an infectious arthritis of an MCP joint does occur, only 10% of the patients will regain their previous level of function and range of motion due to the lack of surgical reconstruction options.[6]

When considering injury to these structures, a noninfectious complication that can occur is simply tendon rupture due to the trauma of the bite itself. Abscess formation can occur, and occasionally infection may spread deep past the periosteum and cause osteomyelitis. It is at this point that these possible complications will be examined. However, a complication that is of significant importance, but is not discussed in this article, includes sepsis with associated bloodstream infection (BSI), as the therapy and diagnostic evaluation for this will be organism specific. An important fact to remember is that *P multocida* BSI has been linked to a 31% mortality rate.[19]

Abscess Formation

Occasionally patients will present with signs and symptoms of an abscess after a bite wound. This may be apparent on physical examination, with a region of fluctuant or indurated skin with associated erythema and edema. If abscess is suspected within deeper muscle or tissue groups, imaging modalities, such as ultrasound, MRI, or computed tomography (CT) may be of utility. Once located, it is paramount to have this evaluated for incision and drainage. In abscesses without other complications, and sufficient drainage, a 7-day course of antibiotics may be sufficient, but this should be reevaluated when nearing the end of therapy to see if an extended course is necessary.

Infectious Arthritis and Tenosynovitis

In patients with bites overlying tendons or joints, the concern for developing infectious arthritis or tenosynovitis should be high. Rapid edema, joint pain, limited mobility, and associated erythema should prompt further imaging and diagnostic evaluation. At this point, it also would be prudent to have the patient evaluated by an orthopedic specialist in the event that debridement or joint incision and drainage are necessary. Blood cultures, and if possible a joint aspiration, should be performed before antibiotic initiation. The joint fluid should be sent for cell count, and cultured. After this is performed, the patient can be started on empiric therapy targeting bacteria listed previously.

Other laboratory studies that may be of utility include an erythrocyte sedimentation rate (ESR) and C-reactive protein (CRP), both of which can be elevated in this setting. Plain radiography may be of limited use, but can evaluate for foreign bodies, such as tooth fragments. MRI of the affected area may reveal joint effusion or abnormalities in the tendon sheath.

Treatment of infectious arthritis will typically involve intravenous antibiotics for a duration of 3 to 4 weeks,[20] whereas tenosynovitis can typically be treated with 7 to 10 days of total therapy.[21] Both of these durations are subject to augmentation based on the predominant organism species and the response to therapy. With good response to intravenous therapy, changing to oral medications to complete the duration is a possibility. In this potential setting, using an antimicrobial agent with good bioavailability, such as a fluoroquinolone, is a good option in combination with one of the anaerobic drugs listed in Table 1, so long as cultures indicate adequate coverage. It is also vital to remember that these patients often will require some physical and occupational therapy once the infection begins to resolve in an attempt to recover as much range of motion as possible of the affected regions.

Osteomyelitis

Depending on the depth of the bite wound, osteomyelitis may be a less-frequent, but potential concern. Cat bites in general should be of higher clinical suspicion due to the previously described difference in dentition, which makes entering bone and joint a more frequent occurrence.[9] In this setting, deep wounds should be evaluated clinically for visualization of exposed bone. It also should be recognized that underlying osteomyelitis secondary to a severely infected skin/soft tissue wound or an infectious arthritis is a possibility due to contiguous spread, and this should be evaluated as a spectrum of disease and not necessarily separate entities. The diagnosis of osteomyelitis can be of higher concern with poor response to therapy in the previously discussed complications and in chronically nonhealing or draining wounds.

Standard laboratory evaluation may be nonspecific and can include abnormalities such as leukocytosis and/or elevated acute-phase reactants (CRP, ESR). Importantly, blood cultures should be drawn. Typically, an MRI of the affected area is the imaging modality of choice to evaluate for osteomyelitis, but if this is not possible, a CT is the alternative test of choice. Occasionally, a triple-phase bone scan may be needed in the setting of surgical hardware being present near the region of concern.[22] A bone biopsy should be performed to establish the diagnosis and to culture the bone fragment for pathogens. This can be performed during debridement of the wound.

The optimal duration for treatment is fundamentally not established, but current guidelines suggest that 4 to 6 weeks of therapy is typically a standard course. These longer durations of therapy are traditionally accepted because it takes approximately 6 weeks for debrided bone to become covered with healthy vascular tissue.[4]

RABIES PROPHYLAXIS

The United States on the whole is considered a low-risk region of the world with regard to the probability of a human contracting rabies. Both cats and dogs are known as being potential vectors worldwide, and this possibility still exists in unvaccinated animals within the United States. Importantly, the most common vectors for transmission in the United States include raccoons, skunks, foxes, and bats.[23] As might be expected, more cats than dogs have been reported as being rabid in the United States due to less strict laws on feline vaccinations and a higher propensity for cats to roam neighborhoods unsupervised.[24]

Potential exposures include the obvious bite wound and also exposure of an open wound or mucous membrane to contaminated saliva. It is recommended that each incident be evaluated on a case-by-case basis with regard to regional epidemiology and if needed it may be necessary to contact your local health department for advice.

In cases in which rabies transmission is a potential concern, one option is to confine and monitor the animal for a period of 10 days. This 10-day period was determined because the virus is active for transmission in the vector's saliva only during a short period when the animal is showing signs of disease. Once these signs develop, the animal will die within this window of time. If the animal lives beyond this period, it is certain that it was not actively shedding the virus at the time of the bite.[24] If the animal becomes sick or dies during this interval, immediate postexposure prophylaxis is needed.[2]

SUMMARY

Bite wounds are quite prevalent in the United States, and prophylactic antibiotics in seemingly uncomplicated, noninfected wounds are required in certain situations. In patients presenting several hours after the inciting bite, infection of the wound is more common. Antimicrobial therapy ought to be directed against typical bacteria found in the biting organism's oral flora, as well as including empiric MRSA coverage in the event the victim has known colonization. Wound cultures can help guide therapy, but broad coverage will often remain a necessity. Amoxicillin/clavulanic acid is the single antibiotic of choice, but various other regimens are available. These wounds can develop significant complications and a thorough physical examination in association with laboratory and imaging diagnostics can help determine the extent of the infection and guide the need for further specialized care. Occasionally, rabies prophylaxis is a concern and each case should be evaluated individually and in collaboration with local health departments.

REFERENCES

1. Nakamura Y, Daya M. Use of appropriate antimicrobials in wound management. Emerg Med Clin North Am 2007;25(1):159–76.
2. Ellis R, Ellis C. Dog and cat bites. Am Fam Physician 2014;90:239–43.
3. Animal bites. World Health Organization. Available at: http://www.who.int/media centre/factsheets/fs373/en/. Accessed May 1, 2016.
4. Mandell GL, Dolin R, Bennett JE. Principles and practice of infectious disease. 7th edition. Philadelphia: Churchill Livingstone Elsevier; 2010.
5. Baddour LM. Soft tissue infections due to dog and cat bites. In: Sexton DJ, editor. UpToDate. Waltham (MA): UpToDate; 2016.
6. Patil P, Panchabhai T, Galwankar S. Managing human bites. J Emerg Trauma Shock 2009;2(3):186.
7. Abrahamian FM, Goldstein EJC. Microbiology of animal bite wound infections. Clin Microbiol Rev 2011;24(2):231–46.
8. Talan DA, Citron DM, Abrahamian FM, et al. Bacteriologic analysis of infected dog and cat bites. N Engl J Med 1999;340(2):85–92.
9. Goldstein EJC. Bite wounds and infection. Clin Infect Dis 1992;14(3):633–40.
10. Talan DA, Abrahamian FM, Moran GJ, et al. Clinical presentation and bacteriologic analysis of infected human bites in patients presenting to emergency departments. Clin Infect Dis 2003;37(11):1481–9.
11. Baddour LM. Soft tissue infections due to human bites. In: Sexton DJ, editor. UpToDate. Waltham (MA): UpToDate; 2016.
12. Endom E. Initial management of animal and human bites. In: Danzl DF, editor. UpToDate. Waltham (MA): UpToDate; 2016.
13. Stevens DL, Bisno AL, Chambers HF, et al. Practice guidelines for the diagnosis and management of skin and soft tissue infections: 2014 update by the Infectious Diseases Society of America. Clin Infect Dis 2014;59(2).
14. McPhee SJ, Papadakis MA, Rabow MW. Current medical diagnosis & treatment 2012. New York: McGraw-Hill Medical; 2012.
15. Smith PF, Meadowcroft AM, May DB. Treating mammalian bite wounds. J Clin Pharm Ther 2000;25(2):85–99.
16. Guay DR. Moxifloxacin in the treatment of skin and skin structure infections. Ther Clin Risk Manag 2006;2(4):417–34.
17. Daum R. Skin and soft-tissue infections caused by Methicillin-Resistant *Staphylococcus aureus*. N Engl J Med 2007;357(13):1357.
18. Goldstein EJC. Comparative in vitro activity of ertapenem and 11 other antimicrobial agents against aerobic and anaerobic pathogens isolated from skin and soft tissue animal and human bite wound infections. J Antimicrob Chemother 2001; 48(5):641–51.
19. Ruddock TL, Rindler JM, Bergfeld WF. *Capnocytophaga canimorsus* septicemia in an asplenic patient. Cutis 1997;60:95–7.
20. Horowitz DL, Horowitz S, Barilla-LaBarca ML. Approach to septic arthritis. Am Fam Physician 2011;84(6):653–60.
21. Sexton DJ. Infectious tenosynovitis. In: Calderwood SB, editor. UpToDate. Waltham (MA): UpToDate; 2016.

22. Pineda C, Espinosa R, Pena A. Radiographic imaging in osteomyelitis: the role of plain radiography, computed tomography, ultrasonography, magnetic resonance imaging, and scintigraphy. Semin Plast Surg 2009;23(02):080–9.

23. Rabies facts & prevention tips. Available at: http://www.americanhumane.org/animals/adoption-pet-care/safety/rabies-facts-prevention.html. Accessed May 1, 2016.

24. Demaria A Jr. When to use rabies prophylaxis. In: Post TW, editor. UpToDate. Waltham (MA): UpToDate; 2016.

A Tale of Two Mononucleosis Syndromes

Cytomegalovirus and Epstein-Barr Virus for the Primary Care Provider

Leah Hampson Yoke, PA-C, MCHS[a,b,*]

KEYWORDS

- Herpes virus • Mononucleosis syndromes • Fevers • Malaise • Pharyngitis
- Splenomegaly • Viremia • Immunocompetent host

KEY POINTS

- Mononucleosis syndromes can present nonspecifically with malaise, fever, and pharyngitis.
- These can be difficult to diagnose in primary care clinics with vague presenting symptoms, laboratory results that can be challenging to interpret, and only supportive treatment as the remedy.
- Epstein-Barr virus (EBV) is the most common virus causing mononucleosis in immunocompetent patients.
- Cytomegalovirus causes severe disease primarily in immunocompromised patients, including those with hematologic malignancies and transplants.
- Heterophile antibody testing is most specific for EBV but can be falsely negative early in the course of infection and falsely positive in inflammatory conditions.

CASE REPORT

A previously healthy 22-year-old man presents to a neighborhood primary care clinic with complaints of malaise, fever, and pharyngitis for the past 3 days. He describes extreme fatigue, and that his neck "feels swollen." Physical examination does indeed show cervical adenopathy with complete blood count (CBC) remarkable for atypical lymphocytosis. A heterophile antibody test is negative.

Disclosure Statement: The author has nothing to disclose.
[a] Vaccine and Infectious Disease Division, Fred Hutchinson Cancer Research Center, 1100 Fairview Avenue North, Mail Stop G4-490, Seattle, WA 98108, USA; [b] Allergy and Infectious Disease Division, University of Washington School of Medicine, 1959 NE Pacific Street, Seattle, WA 98195, USA
* 1100 Fairview Avenue North, Mail Stop G4-490, Seattle, WA 98108.
E-mail address: lyoke@fredhutch.org

INTRODUCTION

Mononucleosis typically describes a constellation of symptoms, including fever, malaise, and pharyngitis. They are common presentations to primary care clinics, yet are often left undiagnosed or misdiagnosed: the differential is broad, the symptoms are nonspecific, and the treatment is often supportive. Even in the immunocompetent patient, however, the sequelae of infection can lead to significant morbidity. This review provides practical information, including evaluation and treatment of mononucleosis syndromes for the primary care provider.

EPSTEIN-BARR VIRUS
Introduction

Primary infection with Epstein-Barr virus (EBV) in the immunocompetent host can cause heterophile-antibody–positive mononucleosis that is characterized most commonly by fever, pharyngitis, and lymphadenopathy. Transferred primarily by saliva, it is known colloquially as the "kissing disease," although in certain populations it can lead to lymphoma, lymphoproliferative disorders, and squamous cell carcinoma.[1]

Pathology and Presentation

EBV infects B cells and the mucosal cells of the nasopharynx. The antibody response to infection is robust, including nonspecific antibodies that can be picked up by the "heterophile antibody" test for use in diagnosis. The immune system provides lifelong control but does not eradicate EBV. If this immunity is significantly impaired, rarely lymphoproliferative disorders or lymphoma can occur.[1]

   Adolescents (10–19 years of age) are most likely to develop symptomatic primary EBV infection.[2–5] The typical incubation period is 30 to 50 days. Presentation can include pharyngitis, fever, and lymphadenopathy. Some patients may present with a diffuse maculopapular rash after the administration of amoxicillin. CBC shows atypical lymphocyte predominance with or without thrombocytopenia.[1,3] Resolution of infection should be within 1 to 3 weeks, although it can take months for the malaise and fatigue to resolve. Chronic mononucleosis (with detectable virus in blood) has uncommonly been described, persisting as long as 6 to 12 months beyond the initial infection.[6] Transmission of EBV is typically through saliva, which is the most infectious bodily fluid and may remain infectious even after the patient is asymptomatic, up to 6 months.[2] EBV also has been isolated in cervical cells and seminal fluid, suggestive of possible sexual transmission.[7,8] The major risk factor for transmission, however, has been found to be via saliva (such as with kissing) due to the high number of viral particles found in saliva.[2,5]

Complications

Splenic rupture
Splenomegaly occurs in approximately 50% of EBV-associated mononucleosis syndromes; splenic rupture is an uncommon but serious complication, occurring in 0.1% to 0.2% of cases.[9,10] Because an enlarged spleen is often palpable in only half of cases and rupture is not always associated with trauma, it is recommended that all patients with confirmed EBV avoid contact sports for at least 3 weeks after presentation.[11] There are case reports of splenic rupture occurring as late as 8 weeks, however, so clinicians should thoroughly carefully counsel patients of the risks associated with contact sports. Interestingly, there is no correlation between hematologic abnormalities, disease severity, and splenic rupture.[9,10,12,13]

Respiratory

In rare cases, extreme swelling of the upper airways secondary to EBV infection can cause respiratory distress and ultimately upper airway obstruction.[12] This is rare and usually in only 1% of cases; however, evaluation for this should occur in the initial visit, including listening for stridor, evaluation of oxygen saturation, and obvious respiratory distress.

Neurologic

EBV infection is associated with neurologic complications, including facial paralysis, Guillain-Barre syndrome, and other meningitic syndromes.[1,14] In patients with significant neurologic symptoms or evidence of such complications, infectious disease consultation is highly recommended.

Rash

A maculopapular rash can be seen with EBV infection, but is more characteristically associated with amoxicillin administration. Traditionally, the rash was reported to have occurred in 95% of patients with amoxicillin exposure due to formation of immune complexes.[12] However, more recent retrospective data suggest the rash is not nearly as common as previously thought. Two studies identify the prevalence of the rash as being 18.5% and 32.9%, respectively[15,16] The rash is not considered an allergic reaction and amoxicillin may be re-trialed.[12,17]

Streptococcus pharyngitis

Streptococcus pharyngitis is a common cause of bacterial pharyngitis and may present similarly or even concurrently with EBV mononucleosis, although estimates of their overlap are unknown. It is recommended that in these cases, testing for Group A *Streptococcus* should be undergone and treatment initiated with antibiotics.[12]

Proliferative disorders

Lymphoma and other proliferative disorders are associated with EBV infections, particularly in certain populations; however, they are out of the scope for discussion within this article.

Testing and Diagnosis

Detection of heterophile antibodies is the main laboratory test used to diagnose EBV infection in the proper clinical context. This test, however, is notoriously insensitive and false negatives are common early in infection. It also can be falsely positive in several inflammatory disease states, including human immunodeficiency virus (HIV), leukemia, lymphoma, and rubella.[18,19] EBV-specific serologies are clinically available laboratory tests, but are not always necessary given that most patients are heterophile antibody positive. However, these serologies may be of value in patients suspected of having infectious mononucleosis but with a discordantly negative heterophile antibody test.

Hoagland criteria are often used for diagnosis and include the following: at least 50% lymphocytes on CBC with 10% being atypical accompanied by fever, adenopathy, and a positive heterophile antibody test. In review of 500 patients with EBV mononucleosis, 100% had lymphadenopathy, with fever and pharyngitis as the next most common symptoms.[20]

Physical examination is somewhat limited in its sensitivity and specificity. In the presence of consistent symptoms, palatine petechiae or posterior auricular, axillary, or inguinal adenopathy increase the likelihood of heterophile antibody positivity. If these physical examination findings are absent, however, the pre-test probability of an EBV mononucleosis is quite low and a heterophile antibody test is unlikely to be helpful.[17]

Streptococcus pharyngitis is common and can present similarly to and even concurrently with EBV mononucleosis. It is recommended that patients with consistent symptoms (those meeting ≥2 of the Centor criteria) be tested for Group A *Streptococcus* and treated accordingly.[12] Primary HIV infection also can present similarly and should not be missed. A review of HIV risk factors and HIV testing, if any are present, should be performed in all patients presenting with fever, malaise, adenopathy, and pharyngitis.[1]

Treatment

The mainstay of care for EBV is supportive, including analgesics, rest, and proper fluid intake. Patients should be counseled against contact sports, as described previously, due to risk of splenic rupture. Patients also should be counseled as to the high transmissibility of EBV through saliva. However, as most of the population is EBV serology positive, this precaution primarily would apply to the immunocompromised or symptomatic. Asymptomatic close contacts do not require serologic testing.[12]

The use of antiviral therapy for EBV within primary care is debated, although a recent review of severe EBV infection in immunocompetent patients suggested that the use of antivirals, most commonly acyclovir, was associated with a favorable outcome.[21] Severe infection included central and peripheral nervous system involvement, hepatitis, respiratory distress, or severe hematologic abnormalities associated with EBV. An infectious disease consultation would be strongly recommended before the consideration of antivirals. Interestingly, in more than half of the cases described, antivirals were used alongside corticosteroids, although their benefit remains unclear.[21] A recent Cochrane database review found insufficient evidence for the use of steroids for symptom control with limited data for long-term efficacy and side effects.[22] However, in specific clinical scenarios, such as impending respiratory obstruction, steroids do have a role and could be a consideration in the appropriate clinical context.

Summary

EBV is an infection commonly seen in primary care offices. Even so, EBV can be challenging to diagnose with inexact laboratory testing combined with a vague clinical syndrome. For the primary care clinician, a constellation of symptoms, including fever, pharyngitis, and adenopathy, with a consistent history should provide sufficient justification to order heterophile antibody testing with concurrent streptococcal throat culture and consideration of HIV testing, dependent on risk. If initial testing is negative but symptoms or laboratory abnormalities persist, the differential should be broadened.

Treatment is supportive, although patients should be counseled regarding risk of splenic rupture. Risk of transmission also should be discussed, although serologic screening tests of asymptomatic contacts are not advised given the high prevalence.

Finally, patients also should be counseled that malaise and fatigue may continue for weeks to months given the perseverance of the virus in the blood stream.

If severe EBV infection is suspected, an infectious disease consultation is highly recommended for the consideration for the use of antivirals. Corticosteroids have shown limited efficacy in the treatment of EBV and should not be used routinely unless under the guidance of an infectious disease consultant.[21]

CYTOMEGALOVIRUS
Introduction

Cytomegalovirus (CMV) is a well-known pathogen in the immune compromised, causing multiple serious complications in transplant recipients and patients with hematologic malignancies. It is a much less common pathogen among the immuno-competent and is therefore often not included in the differential of infectious mono-nucleosis. Among patients with relative immunocompromise, however, including diabetes and rheumatologic disease, primary CMV should be considered.

Pathology

CMV is a double-stranded DNA herpesvirus that in primary infection initially infects mucosal cells, then can infect monocytes and CD34+ stem cells.[23] CMV then estab-lishes a latent state by evasion of the host immune system. The adaptive immune response is primarily responsible for control of this latent phase so any insult to the adaptive response can lead to reemergence of CMV.[23] Reemergence or the reappearance of the virus in blood after initial establishment of latency is termed "reactivation."

Even in a healthy host, CMV is thought to reactivate during times of severe stress. The presence of active or latent CMV may be associated with development of atherosclerosis by causing an inflammatory response in vascular endothelial cells via activation of macrophages and release of inflammatory cytokines and chemokines.[23]

Presentation

Similar to EBV mononucleosis, a patient with primary CMV might present with a nonspecific and self-limiting infection, including fever, pharyngitis, fatigue, and myal-gias accompanied by lymphocytosis. The most common complications include hep-atitis and ampicillin-induced skin rash, which is similar to EBV, along with low-level elevations in liver enzymes.[24–26] Twenty-one percent of mononucleosis syndromes are estimated to be caused by CMV with the remainder due to EBV.[20] There are some distinguishing features, however. Most notably in CMV, fever tends to be the predominant symptom, whereas in EBV, pharyngitis and tonsillar exudates tend to be more common. Transmission is typically via bodily secretions, including via sexual transmission or blood transfusions.[25–27] Due to the high presence of viral particles, however, saliva accounts for most transmission events.

Manifestations in the Immunocompetent

Because manifestations of CMV rarely cause end-organ disease in immunocompetent patients, there is very little literature surrounding this topic. However, some case re-ports have been published describing specifically colitis and uveitis, which are described here.

Gastrointestinal manifestations

Ko and colleagues[28] reported on 51 immunocompetent patients with CMV colitis at a single institution. Based on retrospective analysis, CMV colitis was associated with renal disease, particularly those on hemodialysis, rheumatologic disease, neurologic disease, intensive care unit (ICU) admission, and use of antibiotics, steroids, red blood cell (RBC) transfusions, or antacids. Steroid use and RBC transfusions were consid-ered independent risk factors for developing CMV colitis.[28] Of note, immunocompro-mise was defined as HIV infection, ulcerative colitis, or active cancer; patients with diabetes or active kidney disease were not eliminated from the cohort. An additional caveat of this study is that the seroprevalence of CMV in Korea is higher than in the United States.[28,29]

Goodman and colleagues[30] reviewed published cases of CMV colitis in immunocompetent patients. They reported that even mild immunosuppression, such as in renal disease, can also predispose to CMV infection or reactivation.[30] Although there is no evidence of causative relationship of CMV with inflammatory bowel disease, there is an association. Treatment of the CMV included reduction of immunosuppression. Antiviral agents were used only in severe or refractory disease.[30]

Ocular manifestations
Although most cases of CMV retinitis and uveitis are described in the HIV population, CMV can rarely cause uveitis in the immunocompetent host. In one such case series, the predisposing factor was thought to be intravitreal administration of steroids, emphasizing that the normal immune response is quite effective at controlling CMV.[31]

Critically ill
There are extremely limited data describing immunocompetent patient populations with CMV infections. However, the critically ill patient population with CMV infection is well described, and understanding the principles of CMV infection within this patient cohort can help understand this infection in otherwise immunocompetent patients. In 2009, a meta-analysis was published of patients admitted to an ICU who were CMV serology positive.[32] If admitted more than 5 days, the prevalence of CMV end-organ disease was 36%.[32] Colitis was the most common manifestation of CMV disease in this patient population with mortality reported at nearly 72%, even with antiviral treatment. It was unclear whether CMV reactivation was causative or just a marker of increased mortality risk as described in a similar patient population of critically ill patients.[33]

In 2016, a prospective study was published of CMV seropositive immunocompetent patients. Inclusion criteria included patients who were intubated and mechanically ventilated for more than 4 days.[34] CMV reactivation was associated with increased mortality and was independently associated with case fatality in immunocompetent patients with acute respiratory distress syndrome.[34] It must be noted that some of these patients were receiving high-dose corticosteroids during their ICU stay.

Finally, in an assessment of CMV plasma viremia in a cohort of patients admitted to the ICU, transfusion requirements and diabetes were found to be independent risk factors for CMV reactivation.[35] Reactivation was found to be within 7 days of ICU admission in patients and was associated with elevated inflammatory markers. In addition, sequential organ failure assessment scores were higher in patients with CMV reactivation.[36]

Congenital
Congenital CMV is a very serious complication of primary CMV disease in pregnant women. In developed countries, the rate of congenital CMV infection is 0.6%. This accounts for nearly 40,000 births annually in the United States.[37] Risk factors for maternal and subsequent fetal acquisition of the virus include interaction with young children, young maternal age, and primigravidity.[38] Congenital CMV infection can lead to premature delivery, jaundice, petechial rash, and neurologic complications, including microcephaly, seizures, and poor feeding.[37,39] The most common complication of congenital CMV infection is sensorineural hearing loss, which occurs in approximately 13% of affected infants. Laboratory findings at birth can include

thrombocytopenia and elevated transaminases. The mortality rate of symptomatic infants is 12%.[39]

Testing and Diagnosis

Testing for CMV in an immunocompetent patient includes traditional serology tests with immunoglobulin M suggesting acute infection, although as with EBV, the seroprevalence in the US adult population is quite high. There are approved CMV polymerase chain reaction tests to evaluate the presence of virus in blood and tissue.[26] These tests are most commonly used in immunocompromised patients; however, they may have value in the immunocompetent patient with a non-EBV mononucleosis syndrome.[40]

Summary

CMV is a potential cause of a mononucleosis syndrome in the immunocompetent patient, although it is less commonly a cause of this syndrome than EBV. It can rarely cause end-organ disease, including ocular and gastrointestinal manifestations, although often these patients will have other contributing risk factors. Both as a congenital infection and as an infection in the immunocompromised host, it can cause significant morbidity and mortality. It is important for the primary care provider to be aware of the potential complications of CMV.

DISCUSSION

Primary EBV and CMV both can present as mononucleosis syndromes, although the diagnosis can be challenging for the primary care provider. Based on the higher prevalence of EBV and the lack of definitive treatment in an immunocompetent patient population, a flow chart for diagnosis and treatment is described later in this article. Using evidence-based criteria, if a patient presents between ages 10 and 30 years with adenopathy, pharyngitis, fever, and malaise, consider sending heterophile antibody testing as well as a rapid streptococcus test. HIV also always should be considered in this differential, with testing done if appropriate risk factors are present. If the patient is heterophile antibody test positive, symptomatic treatment is recommended with counseling regarding potential for splenic rupture. Imaging should be avoided unless there is specific concern. If streptococcus rapid test is positive, antibiotics should be given.

Because there is no recommended therapy for a stable patient presenting with an infectious mononucleosis due to CMV, specific diagnostic testing should not be pursued unless there is particular concern for primary CMV, such as in pregnancy or relative immunocompromise. In a recent study, primary care providers reported that using CMV serology for diagnosis was helpful to provide quality care and to avoid further, possibly needless testing.[40] However, ultimately symptomatic treatment is indicated, and in a self-limiting viral syndrome, testing may not be necessary unless symptoms are persistent. In pregnancy, diagnostic testing should be performed if prenatal examinations suggest congenital CMV and with the assistance of obstetric and infectious disease providers.

CMV and EBV are viruses that can cause mononucleosis syndromes with similar presentations. Given potential for significant complications, a diagnostic algorithm (Fig. 1) is helpful in understanding how properly to test and treat these patients in a primary care clinic. Specific patient populations require infectious disease consultations; however, most patients can be managed by a primary care provider with supportive care. Ultimately, an understanding of these 2 mononucleosis syndromes can

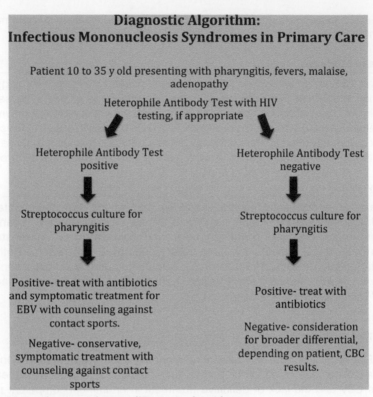

Fig. 1. Mononucleosis syndromes diagnostic algorithm.

lead to better patient care in an outpatient setting with the use of evidence-based methods to accurately diagnose and counsel patients.

REFERENCES

1. Hirsch MS. Herpesvirus infections. In: Singh AK, editor. Infectious disease: the clinician's guide to diagnosis, treatment, and prevention. Decker Publishing Company; 2016. STAT! Ref Online Electronic Medical Library. Available at: http://online.statref.com/offcampus.lib.washington.edu/Documen.aspx?fxId=65&docID=1. Accessed May 31, 2016.

2. Balfour HH Jr, Holman CJ, Hokanson KM, et al. A prospective clinical study of Epstein-Barr virus and host interactions during acute infectious mononucleosis. J Infect Dis 2005;192(9):1505–12.

3. Henke CE, Kurland LT, Elyback LR. Infectious mononucleosis in Rochester, Minnesota: 1950 through 1969. Am J Epidemiol 1973;98(5):483–90.

4. Fry J. Infectious mononucleosis: some new observations from a 15-year study. J Fam Pract 1980;10(96):1087–9.

5. Balfour HH Jr, Odumade OA, Schmeling DO, et al. Behavioral, virologic, and immunologic factors associated with acquisition and severity of primary Epstein-Barr virus infection in university students. J Infect Dis 2013;207(1):80–8.

6. Papesch M, Watkins R. Epstein-Barr virus infectious mononucleosis. Clin Otolaryngol Allied Sci 2001;26(1):3–8.

7. Naher H, Gissmann L, Freese UK, et al. Subclinical Epstein-Barr virus infection of both the male and female genital tract–indication for sexual transmission. J Invest Dermatol 1992;98:791–3.
8. Sixbey JW, Lemon SM, Pagano JS. A second site for Epstein-Barr virus shedding: the uterine cervix. Lancet 1986;2:1122–4.
9. Maki DG, Reich RM. Infectious mononucleosis in the athlete: diagnosis, complications, and management. Am J Sports Med 1982;10(3):162–73.
10. Barlett A, William R, Hiltom M. Splenic rupture in infectious mononucleosis: a systemic review of published case reports. Injury 2016;47(3):531–8.
11. Putukian M, O'Connor FG, Stricker P, et al. Mononucleosis and athletic participation: an evidence based subject review. Clin J Sport Med 2008;18(4):309–15.
12. Luzuriaga K, Sullivan JL. Infectious mononucleosis. N Engl J Med 2010;363(15): 1486.
13. Asgar MM, Begos DG. Spontaneous splenic rupture in infectious mononucleosis: a review. Yale J Biol Med 1997;70(2):175–82.
14. Hughes RA, Hadden RD, Gregson NA, et al. Pathogensis of Guillian-Barre syndrome. J Neuroimmunol 1999;100(1–2):74–97.
15. Hocqueloux L, Guinard J, Buret J, et al. Do penicillins really increase the frequency of a rash when given during Epstein Barr virus primary infection? Clin Infect Dis 2013;57(11):1661–2.
16. Chovel-Sella A, Ben Tov A, Laha E, et al. Incidence of rash after amoxicillin treatment in children with infectious mononucleosis. Pediatrics 2013;131(5):e1424–7.
17. Aronson MD, Komaroff AL, Pass TM, et al. Heterophil antibody in adults with sore throat: frequency and clinical presentation. Ann Intern Med 1982;96(4):505–8.
18. Schumacher HR, Austin RM, Stass SA. False positive serology in infectious mononucleosis. Lancet 1979;1(8118):722.
19. Ebell MH. Epstein-Barr infectious mononucleosis. Am Fam Physician 2004;70(7): 1279–87.
20. Hoagland RJ. Infectious mononucleosis. Prim Care 1975;2(2):295–307.
21. Rafailidis PI, Mavros MN, Kapaskelis A, et al. Antiviral treatment for severe EBV infections in apparently immunocompetent patients. J Clin Virol 2010; 49(3):151–7.
22. Rezk E, Nofal YH, Hamzeh A, et al. Steroids for symptom control in infectious mononucleosis. Cochrane Database Syst Rev 2015;(11):CD004402.
23. La Rosa C, Diamond DJ. The immune response to human CMV. Future Virol 2012; 7(3):279–93.
24. Fiala M, Heiner DC, Turner JA, et al. Infectious mononucleosis and mononucleosis syndromes. West J Med 1977;126(6):445–59.
25. Klemola E, Von Essen R, Henle G, et al. Infectious mononucleosis-like disease with negative heterophile agglutination test. J Infect Dis 1970;121:608–14.
26. Crumpacker CS. Cytomegalovirus. In: Bonnott JE, Dolin R, Dlaser MJ, editors. Mandell, Douglas, and Bennett's principles and practice of infectious disease. 8th edition. Philadelphia: Elsevier; 2015. p. 1738–53.
27. Canterino JE, McCormack M, Gurung A, et al. Cytomegalovirus appendicitis in an immunocompetent host. J Clin Virol 2016;78:9–11.
28. Ko JH, Peck KR, Lee WJ, et al. Clinical presentation and risk factors for cytomegalovirus colitis in immunocompetent adult patients. Clin Infect Dis 2015;60:e20–6.
29. Crespo P, Dias N, Marques N, et al. Gastritis as a manifestation of primary CMV infection in an immunocompetent host. BMJ Case Rep 2015;2015. http://dx.doi.org/10.1136/bcr-2014-206991.

30. Goodman AL, Murray CD, Watkins J, et al. CMV in the gut: a critical review of CMV detection in immunocompetent host with colitis. Eur J Clin Microbiol Infect Dis 2015;34(1):13–8.
31. Radwan A, Metzinger JL, Hinkle DM, et al. Cytomegalovirus retinitis in immuno-competent patients: case reports and literature review. Ocul Immunol Inflamm 2013;21(4):324–8.
32. Kalil AC, Florescu DF. Prevalence and mortality associated with cytomegalovirus infection in non-immunosuppressed patients in intensive care unit. Crit Care Med 2009;37(8):2350–8.
33. Siciliano RF, Castelli JB, Randi BA, et al. Cytomegalovirus colitis in immunocom-petent critically ill patients. Int J Infect Dis 2014;20:71–3.
34. Ong D, Spitoni C, Klouwenberg P, et al. Cytomegalovirus reactivation and mortal-ity in patients with acute respiratory distress syndrome. Intensive Care Med 2016; 42(3):333–41.
35. Roa PL, Perez-Granda MJ, Munoz P, et al. A prospective monitoring study of cytomegalovirus infection in non-immunosuppressed critical heart surgery pa-tients. PLoS One 2015;10(6):e0129447.
36. Frantzeskaki FG, Karampi ES, Kottaridi C, et al. Cytomegalovirus reactivation in general, non-immunosuppressed intensive care unit population: incidence, risk factors, associations with organ dysfunction, and inflammatory biomarkers. J Crit Care 2015;30(2):276–81.
37. Goderis J, Leenheer ED, Smets K, et al. Hearing loss and congenital CMV infec-tion: a systemic review. Pediatrics 2014;135(5):972–82.
38. Pass RF, Hutto C, Ricks R, et al. Increased rate of cytomegalovirus infection among parents of children attending day-care centers. N Engl J Med 1986; 314(22):1414–8.
39. Boppana SB, Pass RF, Britt WJ, et al. Symptomatic congenital cytomegalovirus infection: neonatal morbidity and mortality. Pediatr Infect Dis J 1992;11(2):93–9.
40. Wreghitt TG, Teare EL, Sule O, et al. Cytomegalovirus infection in immunocompe-tent patients. Clin Infect Dis 2003;37(12):1603–6.

Endemic Fungal Infections in the United States

Roy A. Borchardt, PA-C, PhD

KEYWORDS

- Endemic fungi • Endemic mycosis • Coccidioidomycosis • Blastomycosis
- Histoplasmosis • Fungal infections • Treatment • Diagnosis

KEY POINTS

- Endemic mycoses are infections caused by 3 specific fungi, *Blastomyces dermatitidis*, *Coccidioides* spp, and *Histoplasma capsulatum*, mostly found in specific geographic locations of the United States.
- The endemic fungi normally live in the soil and are capable of generating aerosolized spores that, once inhaled into the lungs of humans, can cause infections.
- Endemic mycoses primarily present clinically as mild or asymptomatic pulmonary infections but can progress to more serious pulmonary infections or disseminated disease, especially in immunocompromised hosts.
- Endemic mycoses are often overlooked as a cause of community acquired pneumonia, resulting in delayed antifungal treatment and disease progression or even death.
- Antifungal azoles and amphotericin B are the drugs of choice to treat endemic mycoses, and guidelines are available to help in the medical management of infected patients.

INTRODUCTION

Commonly referred to as the endemic fungi, *Blastomyces dermatitidis*, *Coccidioides* spp, and *Histoplasma capsulatum*, are the 3 primary fungal species that cause endemic mycoses in the United States.[1] All 3 endemic fungi are soil-dwelling microorganisms that are predominantly restricted to specific geographic regions in the United States[2–4]; however, they also can be found to some extent in areas outside traditional endemic regions.[5–7] These endemic fungi are capable of causing a variety of specific diseases in humans but the predominant manifestation is pneumonia.[1,2] The respiratory tract is the main pathway for entry into the human host. Aerosolized spores, released from disrupted soil by activities, such as dust storms, military exercises, and earth excavations, are inhaled into the lungs. Once inside the lungs, the spores

Disclosure Statement: The author has nothing to disclose.
Advanced Practice Providers, Department of Infectious Diseases, Infection Control and Employee Health, MD Anderson Cancer Center, Unit 1460, 1400 Pressler Street, Houston, TX 77030-4009, USA
E-mail address: rborchar@mdanderson.org

Physician Assist Clin 2 (2017) 297–312
http://dx.doi.org/10.1016/j.cpha.2016.12.011
2405-7991/17/© 2016 Elsevier Inc. All rights reserved.

grow and spread to surrounding tissues. The fungi subsequently can spread even further to other tissues of the body by hematological and/or lymphatic routes, and thus can progress to disseminated disease.[1,2] Rarely do infections occur through cutaneous inoculation.[8]

B dermatitidis, *Coccidioides* spp, and *H capsulatum*, cause the specific human endemic fungal infections (endemic mycoses) of blastomycosis, coccidioidomycosis, and histoplasmosis, respectively.[1] Each of these endemic mycoses have specific disease characteristics but they also share some common clinical presentations: (1) the clinical spectrum of disease presentation ranges from asymptomatic to severe life-threatening illness and death, (2) symptomatic disease occurs in both immunocompromised and immunocompetent hosts, and (3) the most common manifestation is pneumonia.[1,2,9] The endemic fungi are frequently overlooked as an underlying cause of community acquired pneumonia.[10] Endemic mycoses can result in hospitalizations and, often in severe cases, can even be fatal. Estimates are that around 10% of all hospitalized cases result in death.[3] In cases of misdiagnosed cause, patients diagnosed with community acquired pneumonia will receive courses of empiric antibacterial therapy without improvement or develop worsening illness before the correct diagnosis of pulmonary endemic mycosis is made and the appropriate antifungal therapy initiated.[10] Delays in diagnosis and proper treatment are the major factors that result in increased morbidity and mortality.

Greater awareness and a more thorough knowledge of the endemic mycoses will likely aid health care providers to better diagnose and treat these illnesses. For all patients who live in or have recently traveled to endemic fungal areas and have suspected community acquired pneumonia, endemic mycosis should be on the differential. Guidelines for the treatment of the endemic mycoses are available through the Infectious Diseases Society of America (see later discussion) but, in general, treatment depends on the severity of the illness and organs affected by the disease. Moreover, 3 excellent reviews on the various endemic mycosis have recently been published[11–13] (see later discussion).

BLASTOMYCOSIS

B dermatitidis is a thermally dimorphic fungus that exists as a mold in the soil and as a yeast in human tissues.[11] It is found primarily in the upper Midwest, southeast, and south-central United States. It is especially endemic to those states bordering the Ohio and Mississippi River Valley but also can be found in northern New York[14] (Fig. 1). The states with the highest number of reported cases of blastomycosis are

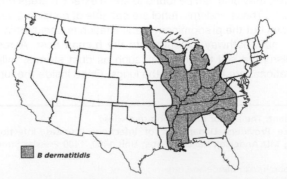

B dermatitidis

Fig. 1. Geographic distribution of *B dermatitidis* in the United States. (*Adapted from* Castillo CG, Kauffman CA, Miceli MH. Blastomycosis. Infect Dis Clin North Am 2016;30:248; with permission.)

Wisconsin, Arkansas, Mississippi, Kentucky, and Tennessee.[11] Cases have been reported for the nontraditional endemic states of Florida, Colorado, and Hawaii.[7] A clustered outbreak was reported for northern Wisconsin, where the incidence was disproportionately higher among Asian residents, in particular among Hmong immigrants. The incidence was 12-fold higher among these people without identifiable higher environmental risk factors. This suggests there is a genetic predisposition to blastomycosis among the Hmong people.[15] B dermatitidis can affect other animals, including dogs.[16] Interestingly, the incidence of blastomycosis among humans is correspondingly high in those areas were its incidence among dogs also is high. One-third of infected people reported their dog also had been diagnosed with blastomycosis.[17]

The main route of infection occurs through inhalation of aerosolized B dermatitidis conidia (asexual spores of the fungi) into the lungs. Once inside the lungs, the conidia convert into the yeast phase in host tissues and spread. An inflammatory response by the host ensues and results in neutrophilic clustering and subsequent formation of noncaseating granulomas with giant cells and epithelioid cells.[11] Primary cutaneous blastomycosis is rare, having been documented to occur after accidental inoculation (in the laboratory or autopsy setting) or from the bite of an infected dog. The incubation period is from 2 to 6 weeks.[18]

Clinical Presentation

Most blastomycosis is asymptomatic or presents as a mild, self-limiting illness.[11,19,20] Symptomatic blastomycosis can present as either an acute or chronic disease. Acute pulmonary blastomycosis symptoms include cough, pleuritic chest pain, fever, chills, and malaise. The cough is initially nonproductive but progresses to productive with purulent sputum. Although uncommon, severe acute pulmonary infection can progress rapidly to adult respiratory distress syndrome (ARDS) in reportedly up to 15% of cases.[11] There is a high mortality, approaching 50%, associated with severe cases of blastomycosis despite appropriate antifungal therapy.[11,19,20] Chronic blastomycosis manifests with persistent productive cough, occasional hemoptysis, fever, night sweats, and weight loss, and is often mistaken for tuberculosis or lung cancer.[11,19,20]

Extrapulmonary blastomycosis is a chronic presentation of disseminated disease that usually occurs in the setting of ongoing pulmonary infection.[11,19,20] B dermatitidis can infect almost every organ of the body. The most common extrapulmonary sites of infection are the skin, bone, and genitourinary system. Skin infection accounts for 60% of all extrapulmonary blastomycosis. Other uncommon sites include the central nervous system (CNS), eyes, uterus, peritoneum, and larynx. The gross and histopathologic appearances of laryngeal blastomycosis can be mistaken for squamous cell carcinoma. Rare instances of human-to-human transmission have been reported for genitourinary blastomycosis causing vaginal and perinatal infections.[11,19,20]

Cutaneous disease is the most common site of extrapulmonary blastomycosis.[19,20] Disseminated cutaneous blastomycosis is unique among the endemic fungal infections with the formation of pseudoepitheliomatous hyperplasia with microabscess formation. The lesions begin as small papulopustules that progress to irregular shaped, raised, verrucous-like crusted nodules or ulcerative nodules, similar in appearance to basal cell carcinoma or squamous cell carcinoma[11,19,20] (Fig. 2).

Skeletal blastomycosis primarily affects the long bones or, less commonly, the vertebrae and ribs. Symptoms more often are the presence of contiguous soft tissue abscesses or sinus tracts but rarely can include localized pain, redness, and increased warmth of overlying tissues. Vertebral blastomycosis can lead to the development of paravertebral or epidural abscess, or can be associated with psoas muscle abscess.[11,19,20]

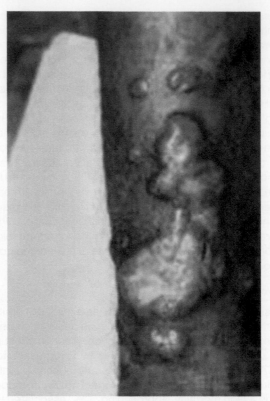

Fig. 2. Cutaneous blastomycosis: skin infection of the arm. (*Courtesy of* CDC/ Dr. Lucille K. Georg, 1971.)

Genitourinary blastomycosis affects men more frequently than women. In men, the prostate is the most common site of genitourinary blastomycosis, followed by testicles and epididymis, with symptoms including dysuria, testicular pain, perineal pain, and urinary obstruction. In women, genitourinary blastomycosis can result in tubo-ovarian and uterine abscess, with progression into the peritoneum, resulting in peritoneal and omental nodules.[11,19,20]

Disseminated blastomycosis can affect the CNS and result in the development of meningitis or brain abscesses. In general, immunocompromised patients, such as individuals with human immunodeficiency virus infection and acquired immune deficiency syndrome (HIV/AIDS), solid organ transplant recipients, hematopoietic stem cell recipients, prolonged glucocorticosteroid recipients, and antitumor necrosis factor alpha (anti-TNF-α) recipients present with more severe symptoms and are more likely to develop respiratory distress that progresses to ARDS in the setting of acute pulmonary blastomycosis.[11,19,20]

Diagnosis

Blastomycosis is readily isolated from respiratory secretions and the definitive diagnosis is made by the isolation of *B dermatitidis* in culture.[19,21] Pulmonary samples can be obtained from sputum or bronchoscopy (culture yields have been reported from 86% to 100%, respectively), and positive cultures will usually grow as an identifiable white mold within 1 to 4 weeks that slowly turns light brown.[19,21] Conversion of the mycelial mold form to the yeast form occurs at 37° centigrade is required for positive identification.[19] Tissue samples positive for *B dermatitidis* can be identified by either culture or direct visualization with histopathological staining and microscopic analysis. A commercial test is available for *Blastomyces* antigen testing of blood, urine, and other fluids.[19,21] The urine antigen has cross-reactivity with *H capsulatum*, so its role in diagnostic testing has yet to be established. Serologic testing is not specific and has low sensitivity, such that its use in routine diagnostic testing is not recommended.[19,21]

Treatment

All persons with blastomycosis with either moderate to severe pneumonia, disseminated infection, or who are immunocompromised should receive antifungal therapy.[11,14] Amphotericin B (amphoB) is used as initial treatment for all patients with severe blastomycosis or with CNS involvement (Box 1). Although earlier clinical

---

Box 1
Treatment of blastomycosis

Mild to moderate blastomycosis

Oral itraconazole with a loading dose 200 mg po tid for 3 days; then itraconazole 200 mg po daily to bid dosing for a total of 6 to 12 months
1. Check itraconazole serum concentrations after 2 weeks or more of therapy to ensure therapeutic levels

Moderately severe to severe blastomycosis

Lipid formulation amphoB at 3 to 5 mg/kg IV per day for 1 to 2 weeks, or until improvement is noted; then either (1) itraconazole therapy or (2) voriconazole therapy for a total of 6 to 12 months for pulmonary blastomycosis and 12 months or more for disseminated extrapulmonary blastomycosis
1. Itraconazole therapy: loading dose of itraconazole 200 mg po tid for 3 days followed by itraconazole 200 mg po bid
    a. Check itraconazole serum concentrations after 2 weeks or more of therapy to ensure therapeutic levels
2. Voriconazole therapy: loading dose of voriconazole 400 mg po bid for 1 day followed by voriconazole 200 mg po bid

CNS blastomycosis

Lipid formulation amphoB at 5 mg/kg IV per day for 4 to 6 weeks, followed by an oral azole for 12 months or more and until resolution of CNS abnormalities with
1. Fluconazole 800 mg po daily; or
2. Itraconazole loading dose 200 mg po tid for 3 days; then, 200 mg po bid to tid; or
3. Voriconazole 200 to 400 mg po bid

Immunosuppressed patients

Lipid formulation amphoB at 3 to 5 mg/kg IV per day for 1 to 2 weeks, or until improvement is noted; then itraconazole loading dose 200 mg po tid for 3 days followed by itraconazole 200 mg po bid for 12 months or more (may require lifelong suppressive therapy if immunosuppression cannot be reversed or with relapse despite appropriate therapy)
1. Check itraconazole serum concentrations after 2 weeks or more of therapy to ensure therapeutic levels

Pregnancy

Avoid azoles in pregnant women; the preferred drug for treatment of blastomycosis in pregnant women is lipid formulation amphoB at 3 to 5 mg/kg IV per day.

Adapted from Chapman SW, Dismukes WE, Proia LA, et al. Clinical practice guidelines for the management of blastomycosis. Clin Infect Dis 2008;46:1801–12.

studies were performed with deoxycholate amphoB, most clinicians now use lipid formulations of amphoB because they have fewer side effects.

Pulmonary blastomycosis
For moderately severe to severe pulmonary blastomycosis, initial treatment is with 1 to 2 weeks lipid amphoB at 3 to 5 mg/kg per day, followed by 6 to 12 months of itraconazole 200 mg by mouth (po) twice a day (bid) after a loading dose of 200 mg po 3 times a day (tid) for 3 days. For immunocompromised patients, initial treatment is with 1 to 2 weeks lipid amphoB at 3 to 5 mg/kg per day, followed by 12 months of itraconazole 200 mg po bid after a loading dose of 200 mg po tid for 3 days. For mild to moderate pulmonary blastomycosis, patients are treated with itraconazole 200 mg po bid for 6 to 12 months after a loading dose of 200 mg po tid for 3 days. The newer generation azoles, voriconazole, posaconazole, and isavuconazole have been used successfully to treat blastomycosis, particularly for refractory disease.[22,23]

Extrapulmonary blastomycosis
For patients with CNS involvement, initial treatment is with 4 to 6 weeks of liposomal amphoB at 5 mg/kg per day (specifically liposomal amphoB because it achieves the highest CNS concentrations in animal models), followed by 12 months or more of an azole with either fluconazole 800 mg po daily, itraconazole 200 mg po bid to tid, or voriconazole 200 to 400 mg po bid. For moderately severe to severe disseminated extrapulmonary blastomycosis, treatment is extended to at least 12 months.

Itraconazole blood concentrations can vary widely among patients receiving treatment, so routine serum concentration monitoring is recommended after steady state levels have been achieved, which is usually around 2 weeks. Voriconazole has been used to treat refractory blastomycosis and as an alternative treatment in CNS blastomycosis. Azoles should be avoided in pregnant women, so the preferred drug to treat blastomycosis in this population is amphoB at 3 to 5 mg/kg per day.[11,14]

There are no clear guidelines to assess the severity of blastomycosis illness; hence, clinical judgment should be used to determine severity.[14] Therefore, obtaining an infectious disease consultation is prudent for optimal patient care because these specialists have the experience and expertise to guide the most appropriate treatment and assess response to therapy.

COCCIDIOIDOMYCOSIS

The *Coccidioides* spp also is a dimorphic fungus that exists as a mycelium in saprobic growth and in parasitic growth as a unique structure called a spherule.[24,25] The mycelia grow just a few inches under the soil, and become fragile and fracture in dry weather, producing 3 to 5 microns diameter spores. The slightest air disturbance will send the spores airborne. The main route of infection occurs through inhalation of aerosolized arthroconidia (fragments of septated hyphal cells) into the lungs. Once inside the lungs, the spores grow into larger 10 to 100 micron diameter structures called spherules that contain multiple 2 to 5 micron diameter endospores. The spherules eventually rupture, sending the endospores into surrounding tissues.[21,25]

There are 2 *Coccidioides* spp, *C immitis* and *C posadasii* that cause coccidioidomycosis.[26] Found primarily in the arid desert regions of the southwestern states of Arizona, California, New Mexico, Nevada, Utah, and West Texas, the *Coccidioides* spp are especially prevalent in the San Joaquin Valley of California and Sonoran desert of Arizona[27] (**Fig. 3**). During the surveillance period from 1998 to 2011, the Centers for Disease Control and Prevention (CDC) reported an 8-fold increased incidence, up from 5.3 per 100,000 in 1998 to 42.6 per 100,000 in 2011. A total of 111,717 cases

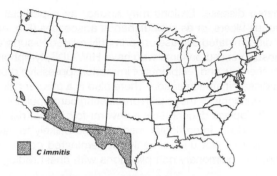

Fig. 3. Geographic distribution of *C immitis* in the United States. (*Adapted from* Castillo CG, Kauffman CA, Miceli MH. Blastomycosis. Infect Dis Clin North Am 2016;30:248; with permission.)

were reported to the CDC during this period, the distribution was such that 66% came from Arizona, 31% from California, 1% from all other endemic states, and less than 1% from nonendemic states.[28] The incidence was increased for all age groups but was highest in people 40 to 59 years old in California, whereas in Arizona and other endemic states it was highest among the 60 years old or older population.[28] Interestingly, Missouri, a state not previously known for endemic coccidioidomycosis, reported a significant increased incidence from 2004 to 2013. The Missouri Department of Health and Senior Services reported an incidence of 0.05 cases per 100,000 in 2004 but increased 5.6-fold to 0.28 per 100,000 in 2013.[6] Of these patients, 48% had traveled to endemic regions of the United States but 26% had not, and the travel history was unknown for the remaining 26%.[6] In 2003, coccidioidomycosis became a reportable disease in Missouri. This change in reporting disease status, coupled with an increased health care provider awareness of the disease and better diagnostic testing, are thought to have contributed to some of the increased incidence but not all.[6] The risk for development of coccidioidomycosis is seasonal, being highest during the dry periods that follow a rainy season.[12]

Clinical Presentation

Most coccidioidomycosis (around 60%) is asymptomatic.[12,25,29] Symptomatic coccidioidomycosis, also known as Valley Fever, can range from a self-limiting influenza-like illness that typically resolves in several weeks to frank pneumonia that may develop into chronic or severe pulmonary disease. Symptoms usually occur 7 to 21 days after exposure. The most common symptoms associated with coccidioidomycosis are fever, cough, and chest pain. Other symptoms may include shortness of breath, hemoptysis, fatigue, lethargy, arthralgia, weight loss, and skin manifestations (nonpruritic fine papular rash; erythema nodosum and erythema multiforme are observed more commonly among women). Patients may develop pulmonary nodules or peripheral thin-walled cavitary lesions on chest imaging. Pleural disease is more common with coccidioidomycosis than with other endemic fungal infections; nonetheless, empyema is a rare manifestation. Less than 1% of infected persons will have disseminated disease. In some severe instances, *Coccidioides* spp may spread into the CNS. The body's response to infection with endospores tends to be neutrophilic inflammation, whereas the response to spherules is generally a granulomatous process. The most common extrapulmonary sites of infection are skin, bone, joints, and the CNS. Cutaneous coccidioidomycosis is the most common form of disseminated disease. Lesions may appear as superficial maculopapules, keratotic or verrucous ulcers, or as subcutaneous abscesses (**Fig. 4**).[12,25,29]

Risk factors for disseminated disease are primarily related to suppression of cellular immunity. Immunosuppressed patients who have HIV/AIDS, lymphoma, solid tumors and receive chemotherapy, and recipients of immunosuppressive drugs are at greater risk of developing disseminated infection. There also is a greater risk for patients with diabetes mellitus, pregnancy, or those with preexisting cardiopulmonary disease. Persons of African or Philippines decent have a several-fold higher risk for disseminated coccidioidomycosis. Adults, in particular men, are more likely to have disseminated disease than are children. Not uncommonly, disseminated coccidioidomycosis will occur in the absence of pulmonary complications with chest radiographs appearing normal.[12,25,29]

Diagnosis

The diagnosis of coccidioidomycosis can be made by the isolation and identification of *Coccidioides* spp spherules from tissue culture. The mold grows slowly, and may take several days or weeks to identify. Positive cultures will develop a nonpigmented white mold colony.[30] Polymerase chain reaction can be used for pulmonary specimens. It has very high sensitivity (100%) and specificity (98%) but sensitivity drops to around 73% in paraffin-embedded tissue specimens. Serologic testing for

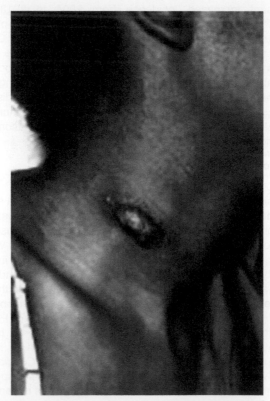

Fig. 4. Cutaneous coccidioidomycosis: chronic neck infection. (*Courtesy of* CDC/ Dr. Lucille K. Georg, 1972.)

Coccidioides immunoglobulin (Ig)-G and IgM with enzyme immunoassay or immuno-diffusion also can be used to help make the diagnosis but false-negative results can occur in up to 38% of samples and there is cross-reactivity in up to 10% of samples with other endemic fungi.[21]

Treatment

Asymptomatic, otherwise healthy, patients with coccidioidomycosis, including those with pulmonary cavities, who do not have significant risk factors for the development of disseminated disease or serious extrapulmonary disease do not need treatment.[2]

Pulmonary coccidioidomycosis

Symptomatic patients are usually treated with an azole or amphoB therapy (Box 2). Common treatment regimens usually start with an oral azole, using either fluconazole 400 mg daily or itraconazole 200 mg bid. The duration of therapy varies according to the severity of the disease but 3 to 6 months is common for uncomplicated pulmonary coccidioidomycosis.

Patients with severe disease or greater risk for disseminated disease, including pregnancy, should be treated. Severity indicators include more than a 10% body weight loss, persistent nights sweats for more than 3 weeks, pulmonary infiltrates involving more than 50% of 1 lung or portions of both lungs, prominent or persistent

---

Box 2
Treatment of coccidioidomycosis

Asymptomatic and pulmonary cavities coccidioidomycosis
  Do not need to treat

Symptomatic, uncomplicated pulmonary coccidioidomycosis
  Oral azole therapy for 3 to 6 months with either fluconazole 400 to 800 mg po daily, or itraconazole 200 mg po bid to tid

Symptomatic, severe pulmonary coccidioidomycosis
  Higher doses azole therapy for 1 year with either po or IV fluconazole 800 to 1000 mg daily, or itraconazole 200 mg po tid, or alternatively,
  Lipid formulation amphoB at 3 to 5 mg/kg IV per day for several weeks until evidence of improvement; then step down to the higher doses azole therapy using either po or IV fluconazole 800 to 1000 mg daily, or itraconazole 200 mg po tid to complete 1 year
1. Monitor the patient every 1 to 3 months for 1 year or longer, to assess for improvement of signs and symptoms, including the establishment of radiographic resolution of the pulmonary infiltrates.

Symptomatic, disseminated nonmeningeal coccidioidomycosis
  Oral azole therapy with either fluconazole 400 to 800 mg po daily or itraconazole 200 mg po bid to tid for 3 to 6 months; for rapidly worsening lesions, lipid formulation amphoB at 3 to 5 mg/kg IV daily for 3 to 6 months

CNS coccidioidomycosis
  Oral azole therapy with either fluconazole 400 to 1000 mg po daily or itraconazole 400 to 600 mg po daily and continued indefinitely if the patient responds to therapy; intrathecal amphoB at 0.1 to 0.5 mg per dose can be added
1. For development of hydrocephalus, a shunt is required for decompression
2. For development of CNS vasculitis, a short course of high-dose IV corticosteroids may help
3. Surgical treatment may be necessary to treat compromise of the vertebral column with associated neurologic deficits.

Adapted from Galgiani JN, Ampel NM, Blair JE, et al. Coccidioidomycosis. Clin Infect Dis 2005;41:1217–23.

hilar adenopathy, anticoccidioidal antibody titers greater than 1:16, inability to work, persistent symptoms for more than 2 months, or age older than 55 years. Higher doses of either intravenous (IV) or oral fluconazole 800 to 1000 mg daily, or oral itraconazole 200 mg tid; or, alternatively, initiation with lipid formulation of amphoB at 3 to 5 mg/kg IV daily with step down to azole therapy after several weeks with evidence for improvement can be used for more severe pulmonary disease. Lipid formulation of amphoB has significant potential side effects of renal toxicity and is expensive but is often used in patients with significant hypoxia or rapid deterioration. Treatment of severe pulmonary disease should continue for at least 1 year. If the patient has severe immunodeficiency, they should remain on an oral azole for secondary prophylaxis. For treatment in pregnancy, amphoB is the preferred therapy due to uncertain fetal safety or potential teratogenic effects of the azoles. For progressive fibrocavitary coccidioidal pneumonia, oral azole is recommended as initial therapy, and continued for 1 year if the patient responds favorably.[2] The newer azoles, voriconazole, posaconazole, and isavuconazole have been used to successfully treat coccidioidomycosis, particularly as salvage therapy when other azoles or amphoB fail.[22,23,31]

Extrapulmonary coccidioidomycosis

For disseminated nonmeningeal coccidioidomycosis, oral azole therapy with either fluconazole 400 to 800 mg daily or itraconazole 200 mg bid to tid can be used. For rapidly worsening lesions, lipid formulations of amphoB at 3 to 5 mg/kg IV daily are warranted. Treatment is usually for 3 to 6 months.[2] For disseminated coccidioidomycosis involving the CNS, azole therapy with either fluconazole 400 to 1000 mg daily or itraconazole 400 to 600 mg daily should be used and continued indefinitely if the patient responds to therapy. Intrathecal amphoB at 0.1 to 0.5 mg per dose can be added. For patients who develop hydrocephalus, a shunt is required for decompression. Coccidioidal meningitis may cause life-threatening cerebral ischemia, infarction, or hemorrhage. A short course of high-dose IV corticosteroids may help for CNS vasculitis.[2] Surgical treatment may be necessary for infection that compromises the vertebral column and causes neurologic deficits.[12]

Patients with severe pulmonary coccidioidomycosis or disseminated disease should be monitored every 1 to 3 months for at least 1 year, or longer, to assess for improvement of signs and symptoms and, in the case of pulmonary coccidioidomycosis, establishment of radiographic resolution of the pulmonary infiltrates. Assessment should include serial serologic testing because increasing *Coccidioides* antibody titers may imply disease progression or evolving dissemination. The interval between visits can be decreased to every 3 to 6 months after establishment of disease improvement.[2] Obtaining an infectious disease consultation will help ensure that patients with coccidioidomycosis receive optimal care because these specialists have the experience and expertise to guide the most appropriate treatment and monitor the response to therapy.

HISTOPLASMOSIS

H capsulatum is endemic to the Midwest and southeastern United States, especially in the Ohio and Mississippi River Valley.[13,32] Histoplasmosis is probably the most common endemic fungal infection in the United States[33] (Fig. 5). *H capsulatum* grows very well in decaying organic rich soil that has been enriched by bird or bat droppings.[13,32] *H capsulatum* is another thermally dimorphic fungus that exists as a mold in the soil and as a yeast in human tissues.[13,32] Infection occurs after high inoculum exposure from activities such as demolition of old buildings; cleaning buildings, such as chicken coups, attics, or barns; cave exploration; and following soil excavation.[13,32–34] The

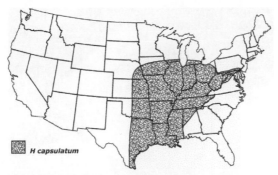

Fig. 5. Geographic distribution of *H capsulatum* in the United States. (*Adapted from* Castillo CG, Kauffman CA, Miceli MH. Blastomycosis. Infect Dis Clin North Am 2016;30:248; with permission.)

main route of infection occurs through inhalation of aerosolized *H capsulatum* microconidia (small spores) into the lungs.[13,32–34] Once inside the lungs, the microconidia are phagocytosed by resident macrophages where they convert into the yeast phase, an essential pathogenic step before they can spread to other tissues.[32] *H capsulatum* is an intracellular pathogen.[32] The phagocytized microconidia and yeast survive inside the macrophages and can disseminate to other tissues as the macrophages travel through the lymphatic system.[13,32–34] Disseminated disease can occur in immunocompromised patients with T-cell deficiencies such as HIV/AIDS, hematological malignancies, solid organ transplant recipients, or patients who receive immunosuppressive drugs such as anti-TNF-α or high-dose steroids.[13,32]

Clinical Presentation

Most cases of histoplasmosis are asymptomatic or have a mild influenza-like illness with low inoculum exposure and can last for more than 1 month.[13,32] Symptomatic disease presents with fever, headache, nonproductive cough, chills, sweats, malaise, and chest pain occurring 1 to 3 weeks after high inoculum exposure. Severe cases can result in respiratory failure and death. Chest radiographic imaging may reveal lobar or patchy pulmonary infiltrates.[13,32] Histoplasmosis is the most commonly diagnosed endemic fungal infection in the United States and is responsible for most hospitalization due to endemic mycoses.[3,33]

Disseminated histoplasmosis can affect any tissue of the body and is capable of causing mediastinitis, hepatosplenomegaly, extrapulmonary lymphadenopathy, oral lesions, skin lesions, adrenal masses, or intestinal masses.[13,32] Usually, disseminated disease occurs in the gastrointestinal (GI) tract, liver, spleen, bone marrow, and skin (Fig. 6). In severe cases, *H capsulatum* can spread to the CNS. Disseminated histoplasmosis is an AIDS-defining illness and, in endemic areas, often is the first symptomatic manifestation of AIDS.[13,32] In the immunocompromised HIV-infected patient with low CD4 count, left untreated, disseminated histoplasmosis is universally fatal.[35]

Diagnosis

The diagnosis of histoplasmosis can be made by the isolation and identification of *H capsulatum* microconidia (3–5 microns diameter) and macroconidia (8–15 microns diameter) from the culture of any tissue.[21,32] The mold grows slowly and may take from to 1 to 6 weeks to identify in culture as a white or brown colony. Serologic testing for the *H capsulatum* antibody can be performed but is less sensitive in

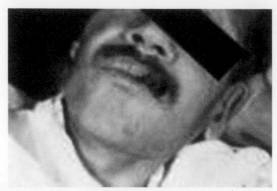

Fig. 6. Cutaneous histoplasmosis: upper lip skin ulcerative infection. (*Courtesy of* CDC/ Susan Lindsley, VD, 1973.)

immunocompromised HIV patients (50%–70%) than in immunocompetent patients (90%).[21,32] Moreover, false-positive results can be seen in patients with tuberculosis, lymphoma, and other endemic fungal infections, especially blastomycosis. The *H capsulatum* antigen can be detected in urine (95%–100% sensitivity), serum (92%–100% sensitivity), or bronchoalveolar lavage (93% sensitivity) by a third-generation polyclonal enzyme immunosorbent assay but still has cross-reactivity with several other fungi, including *Blastomyces* and *Coccidioides* spp.[21,32]

Treatment

Persons with pulmonary histoplasmosis, disseminated disease, CNS involvement, or those who are immunocompromised should receive antifungal therapy.[36] The efficacy of antifungal treatment is uncertain or not recommended for persons with mediastinal disease, inflammatory syndromes (pericarditis, arthritis, and erythema nodosum), pulmonary nodule, broncholithiasis, or ocular histoplasmosis syndrome. Mild pericardial histoplasmosis, mediastinal lymphadenitis histoplasmosis, mediastinal granulomatous histoplasmosis, and pulmonary nodules (histoplasmomas) do not require antifungal therapy and can be treated with nonsteroidal anti-inflammatory drugs.[36]

Pulmonary histoplasmosis

For moderately severe to severe pulmonary histoplasmosis, the initial treatment is with lipid amphoB at 3 to 5 mg/kg per day (add methylprednisolone 0.5–1 mg/kg IV daily for the first 1–2 weeks of antifungal therapy for patients who develop respiratory distress or hypoxia), followed by a load of itraconazole 200 mg po tid for 3 days; then 200 mg PO bid to complete 12 weeks total (Box 3). For mild to moderate pulmonary histoplasmosis with symptoms for more than 4 weeks, recommended treatment is to load with itraconazole 200 mg po tid for 3 days; then 6 to 12 weeks of itraconazole 200 mg po once daily or bid. For mild to moderate pulmonary histoplasmosis with symptoms lasting less than 4 weeks, no treatment is indicated.

Extrapulmonary histoplasmosis

For histoplasmosis with CNS involvement, treatment consists of liposomal amphoB at 5 mg/kg per day for 4 to 6 weeks, followed by at least 12 months of itraconazole 200 mg po bid. Chronic cavitary pulmonary histoplasmosis should be treated with itraconazole 200 mg po tid for 3 days; then 200 mg PO bid for at least 12 months (some clinicians recommend treating for 18–24 months to prevent relapse). Moderate to

Box 3
Treatment of histoplasmosis

Mediastinal histoplasmosis, inflammatory histoplasmosis syndromes (pericarditis, arthritis, and erythema nodosum), solitary histoplasmosis pulmonary nodule, histoplasmosis broncholithiasis, or ocular histoplasmosis syndrome
    Antifungal treatment usually unnecessary; treatment with nonsteroidal anti-inflammatory agents may be prescribed

Mild to moderate acute pulmonary histoplasmosis
    For symptoms for 4 weeks or less, no need to treat
    For symptoms for 4 weeks or more, oral itraconazole with a loading dose 200 mg po tid for 3 days; then itraconazole 200 mg po daily to bid dosing for 6 to 12 weeks

Moderately severe to severe pulmonary histoplasmosis
    Lipid formulation amphoB at 3 to 5 mg/kg IV per day for 1 to 2 weeks, followed by a loading dose of itraconazole 200 mg po tid for 3 days; then, itraconazole 200 mg po bid for a total of 12 weeks
1. Add methylprednisolone 0.5 to 1 mg/kg IV daily for the first 1 to 2 weeks of antifungal therapy if respiratory distress or hypoxia occur

Chronic cavitary pulmonary histoplasmosis
    Oral itraconazole with a loading dose 200 mg po tid for 3 days; then itraconazole 200 mg po Daily to bid dosing for at least 12 months
1. Some experts recommend treating for 18 to 24 months to prevent relapse

Moderately severe to severe pericardial histoplasmosis
    Oral itraconazole with a loading dose 200 mg po tid for 3 days; then, itraconazole 200 mg po daily to bid dosing for 6 to 12 weeks, and
    Add prednisone 0.5 to 1 mg/kg daily and taper down over 1 to 2 weeks; add prednisone 0.5 to 1 mg/kg daily and taper down over 1 to 2 weeks

Disseminated histoplasmosis
    Mild to moderate: oral itraconazole with a loading dose 200 mg po tid for 3 days; then itraconazole 200 mg po bid for at least 12 months
    Moderate to severe: lipid formulation amphoB with either liposomal amphoB at 3 mg/kg IV per day, or lipid complex amphoB at 5 mg/kg IV daily for 1 to 2 weeks, followed by a loading dose of itraconazole 200 mg po tid for 3 days; then itraconazole 200 mg po bid for at least 12 months
1. Measure serum and urine *H capsulatum* antigen levels during and for 12 months after completion of antifungal therapy

CNS histoplasmosis
    Lipid formulation amphoB at 5 mg/kg IV per day for 4 to 6 weeks, followed by a loading dose of itraconazole 200 mg po tid for 3 days; then itraconazole 200 mg po bid for at least 12 months.

Immunocompromised patients
    If immunosuppression cannot be reversed, lifelong suppressive therapy with itraconazole 200 mg PO daily may be necessary

Pregnancy
    Avoid azoles, use lipid formulation amphoB at 3 to 5 mg/kg IV daily for 4 to 6 weeks

Children
    AmphoB deoxycholate is well tolerated at 1 mg/kg IV daily; itraconazole dose is 5 to 10 mg/kg daily in 2 divided doses, do not to exceed 400 mg daily.

Adapted from Wheat LJ, Freifeld AG, Kleinman MB, et al. Clinical practice guidelines for the management of patients with histoplasmosis: 2007 update by the Infectious Diseases Society of America. Clin Infect Dis 2007;45:807–25.

severe pericardial histoplasmosis is treated with itraconazole 200 mg po once daily or bid for 6 to 12 weeks, plus prednisone 0.5 to 1 mg/kg daily tapered down over 1 to 2 weeks. For moderate to severe disseminated histoplasmosis, the treatment is lipid amphoB with either liposomal amphoB at 3 mg/kg per day, or lipid complex amphoB at 5 mg/kg IV daily for 1 to 2 weeks, followed by a loading dose of itraconazole 200 mg po tid for 3 days; then at least 12 months of itraconazole 200 mg po bid. Mild to moderate disseminated histoplasmosis should be treated with a loading dose of itraconazole 200 mg po tid for 3 days; then at least 12 months of itraconazole 200 mg po bid. *H capsulatum* antigen in serum and urine should be measured during and 12 months after completion of therapy for patients with disseminated histoplasmosis. For immunocompromised patients, for whom immunosuppression cannot be reversed, lifelong suppressive therapy with itraconazole 200 mg po daily may be necessary. Itraconazole suspensions are much better absorbed from the GI tract than the tablet formulation.[36]

Other treatment considerations
For histoplasmosis in pregnant women, azoles should not be used. Instead, use lipid amphoB at 3 to 5 mg/kg IV daily for 4 to 6 weeks. For children, acute pulmonary histoplasmosis is common, whereas chronic pulmonary histoplasmosis has not been described. Children also are more likely to experience airway obstruction from mediastinal lymphadenitis histoplasmosis due to more pliable airways than in adults. Unlike adults, children tolerate amphoB deoxycholate well at 1 mg/kg IV daily. The itraconazole dose for children is 5 to 10 mg/kg daily in 2 divided doses (not to exceed 400 mg daily).[36]

Other azoles can be used to treat histoplasmosis.[22,23] Voriconazole has good activity against *H capsulatum* in vitro and has been used successfully to treat histoplasmosis.[22] Posaconazole has very good activity against *H capsulatum* in vitro and has been used successfully to treat histoplasmosis.[22] Recently, isavuconazole has been reported to be successful in the treatment of histoplasmosis.[23] Fluconazole is well tolerated but is inactive against *H capsulatum* in vitro. The Mycoses Study Group reported successful treatment of chronic pulmonary histoplasmosis in only 45% of patients treated with fluconazole.[37] Fluconazole treatment of histoplasmosis has been demonstrated to lead to the development of resistance in AIDS patients. Consequently, fluconazole is not recommended as standard treatment of histoplasmosis and should only be used for those who cannot achieve good therapeutic blood levels with or are intolerant of itraconazole.[36] As with the other endemic fungal infections, obtaining an infectious disease consultation will help ensure that patients with histoplasmosis receive the most appropriate care because these specialists have the experience and expertise in identifying the optimal treatment plan and monitoring the response to therapy.

SUMMARY

The 3 endemic fungi, *B dermatitidis*, *Coccidioides* spp, and *H capsulatum*, are soil-dwelling microorganisms distributed over specific regions of the United States. These fungi cause the endemic mycoses of blastomycosis, coccidioidomycosis, and histoplasmosis. Clinically, these can present as a variety of specific tissue infections but primarily as pneumonia. The respiratory tract is the main pathway for entry into the human host as aerosolized spores are inhaled into the lungs. The fungal spores grow in the lungs and can spread to other tissues of the body causing disseminated disease.

The endemic fungi are a frequently overlooked cause of community acquired pneumonia. Misdiagnosis delays initiation of appropriate antifungal therapy with potentially devastating consequences for the patient, including death. The Infectious Diseases Society of America has evaluated and rated the quality of evidence in published literature for the treatment of the endemic mycoses. Their recommendations for treatment are published and can be found via the following link: http://www.idsociety.org/ Organism/. Under "Infections by Organism," click on the "+Fungi" option to open up to the various guidelines. The guidelines can be accessed by clicking on the hyperlinks, "Link to full-text guideline," or by downloading the individual guideline PDFs. For convenience, the specific PDF links include

Blastomycosis: http://cid.oxfordjournals.org/content/46/12/1801.full.pdf+html
Coccidioidomycosis: http://cid.oxfordjournals.org/content/41/9/1217.full.pdf+html
Histoplasmosis: http://cid.oxfordjournals.org/content/45/7/807.full.pdf+html.

REFERENCES

1. Pfaller MA, Diekema DJ. Epidemiology of invasive mycoses in North America. Crit Rev Microbiol 2010;36(1):1–53.
2. Galgiani JN, Ampel NM, Blair JE, et al. Coccidioidomycosis. Clin Infect Dis 2005; 41:1217–23.
3. Chu JH, Feudtner C, Heydon K, et al. Hospitalizations for endemic mycoses: a population-based national study. Clin Infect Dis 2006;42:822–5.
4. Baddley JW, Winthrop KL, Patkar N, et al. Geographic distribution of endemic fungal infections among older persons, United States. Emerg Infect Dis 2011; 17(9):1664–9.
5. Litvintseva AP, Marsden-Haug N, Hurst S, et al. Valley fever: finding new places for an old disease: *Coccidioides immitis* found in Washington state soil associated with recent human infection. Clin Infect Dis 2015;60:e1–3.
6. Turabelidze G, Aggu-Sher RK, Jahanpour E, et al. Coccidioidomycosis in a state where it is not known to be endemic – Missouri, 2004-2013. MMWR Morb Mortal Wkly Rep 2015;64(23).636–9.
7. Benedict K, Thompson GR, Deresinski S, et al. Mycotic infections acquired outside areas of known endemicity, United States. Emerg Infect Dis 2015; 21(11):1935–41.
8. Smith JA, Riddell J, Kaufamn CA. Cutaneous manifestations of endemic mycoses. Curr Infect Dis 2013;15(2):440–9.
9. Miller R, Assi M, AST Infectious Diseases Community Practice. Endemic fungal infections in solid organ transplantation. Am J Transplant 2013;13:250–61.
10. Hage CA, Know KS, Wheat LJ. Endemic mycoses: overlooked causes of community acquired pneumonia. Respir Med 2012;106:769–76.
11. Castillo CG, Kauffman CA, Miceli MH. Blastomycosis. Infect Dis Clin North Am 2016;30:247–64.
12. Stockamp NW, Thompson GR. Coccidioidomycosis. Infect Dis Clin North Am 2016;30:229–46.
13. Wheat LJ, Azar MM, Bahr NC, et al. Histoplasmosis. Infect Dis Clin North Am 2016;30:207–27.
14. Chapman SW, Dismukes WE, Proia LA, et al. Clinical practice guidelines for the management of blastomycosis. Clin Infect Dis 2008;46:1801–12.
15. Roy M, Benedict K, Deak E, et al. A large community outbreak of blastomycosis in Wisconsin with geographic and ethnic clustering. Clin Infect Dis 2013;57:655–62.
16. Saccente M, Woods GL. Clinical and laboratory update on blastomycosis. Clin Microbiol Rev 2010;23:367–81.

17. Baumgardner DJ, Buggy BP, Mattson BJ, et al. Epidemiology of blastomycosis in a region of high endemicity in north central Wisconsin. Clin Infect Dis 1992;15: 629–35.

18. Gray NA, Baddour CM. Cutaneous inoculation blastomycosis. Clin Infect Dis 2002;34:e44–9.

19. Chapman SW. *Blastomyces* dermatitidis. In: Mandel GL, Bennett JE, Dolin R, editors. Principles and practice of infectious diseases. 6th edition. vol. 2. Philadelphia: Elsevier Churchill Livingstone; 2005. p. 3026–40. Chapter 263.

20. Lopez-Martinez R, Mendez-Tovar LJ. Blastomycosis. Clin Dermatol 2012;30: 565–72.

21. Guarner J, Brandt ME. Histopathologic diagnosis of fungal infections in the 21st century. Clin Microbiol Rev 2011;24(2):247–80.

22. Freifeld AG, Bariola JR, Andes D. The role of second-generation antifungal triazoles for treatment of endemic mycoses. Curr Infect Dis Rep 2010;12:471–8.

23. Thompson GR, Rendon A, Ribiero dos Santos R, et al. Isavunconazole treatment of Cryptococcosis and dimorphic mycoses. Clin Infect Dis 2016;63:356–62.

24. Nguyen C, Barker BM, Hoover S, et al. Recent advances in our understanding of the environmental, epidemiological, immunological, and clinical dimensions of coccidioidomycosis. Clin Microbiol Rev 2013;26:505–25.

25. Galgiani J. *Coccidioides* species. In: Mandel GL, Bennett JE, Dolin R, editors. Principles and practice of infectious diseases. 6th edition. vol. 2. Philadelphia: Elsevier Churchill Livingstone; 2005. p. 3040–51. Chapter 264.

26. Brown J, Benedict K, Park BJ, et al. Coccidioidomycosis: epidemiology. Clin Epidemiol 2013;5:185–97.

27. Galgiani JN. Coccidioidomycosis: a regional disease of national importance – rethinking approaches to control. Ann Intern Med 1999;130:293–300.

28. Tang CA, Tabnak F, Vugia DJ, et al. Increase in reported coccidioidomycosis – United States, 1998-2011. MMWR Morb Mortal Wkly Rep 2013;62(12):217–21.

29. Saubolle MA, McKellar PP, Sussland D. Epidemiologic, clinical, and diagnostic aspects of coccidioidomycosis. J Clin Microbiol 2007;45:26–33.

30. Malo J, Luraschi-Monjagatta C, Wold DM, et al. Update on the diagnosis of pulmonary coccidioidomycosis. Ann Am Thorac Soc 2014;11(2):243–53.

31. Kim MM, Vikram HR, Kusne S, et al. Treatment of refractory coccidioidomycosis with Voriconazole or posaconazole. Clin Infect Dis 2011;53:1060–6.

32. Deepe GS Jr. *Histoplasma capsulatum*. In: Mandel GL, Bennett JE, Dolin R, editors. Principles and practice of infectious diseases. 6th edition. vol 2. Philadelphia: Elsevier Churchill Livingstone; 2005. p. 3012–26. Chapter 262.

33. Benedict K, Mody RK. Epidemiology of histoplasmosis outbreaks, United States, 1938-2013. Emerg Infect Dis 2016;22(3):370–8.

34. Kaufman CA. Histoplasmosis: a clinical and laboratory update. Clin Microbiol Rev 2007;20:115–32.

35. Adenis AA, Aznar C, Couppie P. Histoplasmosis in HIV-infected patients: a review of new developments and remaining gaps. Curr Trop Med Rep 2014;1:119–28.

36. Wheat LJ, Freifeld AG, Kleinman MB, et al. Clinical practice guidelines for the management of patients with histoplasmosis: 2007 update by the Infectious Diseases Society of America. Clin Infect Dis 2007;45:807–25.

37. McKinsey DS, Kauffman CA, Pappas PG, et al. Fluconazole therapy for histoplasmosis. Clin Infect Dis 1996;23:996–1001.

Hepatitis C

An Update on Next Generation Treatment and Clinical Cure

Erin DuHaime, PA-C

KEYWORDS

- Chronic hepatitis C • Hepatitis C treatment • Hepatitis C virus • Antiviral therapies
- Direct-Acting antivirals • Sustained virologic response

KEY POINTS

- Hepatitis C is an important chronic infectious disease that has been historically difficult to treat with regimens that were difficult to tolerate and had poor efficacy.
- Now, with the introduction of new antiviral therapies for hepatitis C virus, there are regimens with markedly improved tolerability and dosing schedules and efficacy for all genotypes.
- It is important for providers to be familiar with the risk factors and screening guidelines/recommendations for hepatitis C.

INTRODUCTION

With regard to hepatitis C disease, it is an exciting time to practice medicine, particularly infectious disease, gastroenterology, hepatology and even primary care, as clinicians are finally able to offer patients who are chronically infected with hepatitis C virus (HCV) a clinical cure. For years, there were limited choices for hepatitis C therapy, with regimens that were ultimately difficult to tolerate and ineffective at achieving a sustained virologic response (SVR), or cure. Now, with the introduction of new antiviral therapies for hepatitis C, there are regimens with markedly improved tolerability and dosing schedules and efficacy approaching 100% for all genotypes.

ETIOLOGY

Hepatitis C is a disease caused by HCV, a spherical, enveloped, single-stranded RNA virus, approximately 9600 nucleotides in length, belonging to the family Flaviviridae, which is further divided into 3 genera: *Flavivirus*, *Pestivirus*, and *Hepacivirus*.

Disclosure Statement: On speakers Bureau for AbbVie.
North Texas Infectious Diseases Consultants, Baylor University Medical Center, 3409 Worth Street, Suite 710, Dallas, TX 75246, USA
E-mail address: erin.duhaime@ntidc.org

Physician Assist Clin 2 (2017) 313–326
http://dx.doi.org/10.1016/j.cpha.2016.12.012   **physicianassistant.theclinics.com**

Flaviviruses include yellow fever virus, dengue fever virus, Japanese encephalitis virus, and tick-borne encephalitis virus. *Pestiviruses* include bovine viral diarrhea virus, classical swine fever virus, and Border disease virus. HCV is a member of the *Hepacivirus* genus, which also includes tamarin virus and GB virus B and is closely related to human virus GB virus C.[1–3]

There are 6 major hepatitis C genotypes and more than 50 subtypes, which differ on a molecular level, including 1a, 1b, 2a, 2b, 3a, 3b, 4, 5, and 6. Although genotype 1 is the most common genotype found worldwide, HCV genotypes have a well-defined geographic distribution. Genotype 1 is most commonly found in the United States, Latin America, and Europe (2 and 3 are less commonly found, and 4, 5, and 6 are rare in these areas). Genotype 3 is most commonly found in India, Southeast Asia/ Indonesia and Australia, and genotype 4 is most commonly found in Africa and the Middle East. Genotype 5 is the predominating HCV genotype in South Africa, whereas genotype 6 predominates in Southeast Asia (**Fig. 1**).[1,4,5]

Determining the HCV genotype is fundamental in treatment planning, as the response to antiviral therapy, dosing, and duration all depend on the genotype. Additionally, the genotype can indicate the rate of disease progression.[6] For example, genotype 1 is thought to have quicker disease progression to cirrhosis and hepatocellular carcinoma (HCC) and was traditionally more difficult to treat, whereas genotype 2 and 3 were typically most responsive to therapy. The emergence of new antiviral regimens, however, has leveled the playing ground, making treatment and clinical cure a possibility, despite the genotype.

PATHOPHYSIOLOGY

After transmission via blood-borne exposure, HCV enters the bloodstream and primarily infects the hepatocytes of the liver, replicating thru a complex series including viral attachment, entry, and fusion via endocytosis, translation of the HCV RNA genome, polyprotein processing, replication, viral assembly, and release. HCV replicates quickly within the cytoplasm of the cell, producing trillions of new viral particles daily, causing detectable viremia.[7,8] HCV replication is accomplished using HCV-specific proteins and enzymes (envelope proteins E1/2, nonstructural proteins NS2, NS3, NS4A, NS4B, NS5A, NS5B, and polypeptide p7 of note), many of which are used as targets of new direct-acting antiviral agents (**Fig. 2**).[9]

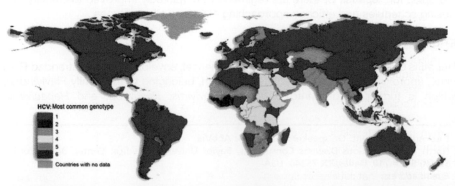

Fig. 1. World distribution of HCV genotypes. (*From* Messina JP, Humphreys I, Flaxman A, et al. Global distribution and prevalence of hepatitis C virus genotypes. Hepatology 2015;61:82; with permission.)

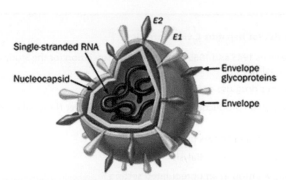

Fig. 2. Hepatitis C virus. (*From* Johns Hopkins Hospital Division of Gastroenterology & Hepatology. Viral Hepatitis C: Introduction. Available at: https://www.jhmicall.org/GDL_Disease. aspx?CurrentUDV=31&GDL_Disease_ID=F90D3628-F21C-41B8-873E-FFFD82A8AF4C&GDL_DC_ID=9AA60584-3607-4D15-A459-BD3F67A3A4A7)

TRANSMISSION AND RISK FACTORS

As mentioned above, HCV is transmitted through blood exposure from an infected source. Those at risk for HCV include IV drug users (past or current); recipients of donated blood, blood products, and organs before 1992; recipients of clotting factors made before 1987; people who required hemodialysis; people who received body piercing or tattoos performed with potentially nonsterile instruments; and people exposed to the blood of someone who tested positive for HCV, via unprotected sexual contact, vertical transmission, occupational exposure, or sharing razors or toothbrushes for example.[4,10]

EPIDEMIOLOGY

The Centers for Disease Control and Prevention reports an estimated 3 to 4 million people in the United States and an estimated 170 million people in the world have chronic hepatitis C disease.[10] Most of those living with HCV are asymptomatic, and a large number of those cases are undiagnosed (cited to be upwards of 50%).[6,10] Routine screening of high-risk patients would not only aide in the diagnosis and treatment of this undiagnosed patient population but also help decrease the transmission rates globally and, therefore, decrease HCV-related morbidity and mortality. Although the recommendations vary slightly between the Centers for Disease Control and Prevention,[10] American Association for the Study of Liver Disease (AASLD)/Infectious Diseases Society of America (IDSA),[6] and the National Institutes of Health,[11] all organizations recommend screening for HCV routinely in those groups at higher risk for infection, including those patients (Box 1).

The frequency of screening for hepatitis C depends on the risk. For example, a one-time screening would be appropriate if their risk is based on birth year; however, more frequent screening may be indicated if the patient participates in high-risk activities, such as intravenous drug use or unprotected sex with numerous partners of unknown human immunodeficiency virus (HIV) or HCV status.[10] HCV screening once annually is recommended for intravenous drug users and men who have sex with men who are HIV-positive, for example.

Considering that routine screening with an HCV antibody test is a cost effective and efficient tool that can be easily added to most laboratory panels, the real question is, what opportunities do providers have for HCV screening? Primary care providers and gastroenterologists, for example, have ample opportunity to routinely screen, for

> **Box 1**
> **Groups at higher risk for hepatitis C virus infection**
>
> Born between the years 1945 and 1965 (per American Association for the Study of Liver Disease, regardless of nationality)
>
> History of intravenous drug use or intranasal drug use
>
> History of receiving blood products/organs before July 1992 (per National Institutes of Health, before 1990)
>
> History of receiving clotting factors made before 1987
>
> History of requiring chronic hemodialysis
>
> History of receiving a tattoo in an unregulated setting
>
> History of incarceration
>
> History of multiple sex partners
>
> HIV positivity
>
> Evidence of liver disease
>
> Had an occupational exposure to blood products
>
> Been born to an HCV-positive woman
>
> Been considered to be a solid organ donor
>
> *Data from* Refs.[6,10,11]

instance, at an annual physical or during an office visit when a patient presents for sexually transmitted disease testing or before a screening colonoscopy. These are not official recommendations of any organization; however, they are examples of the screening opportunities available to providers in everyday practice.

Looking forward, as providers start initiating and enforcing the screening guidelines, the incidence of hepatitis C disease may increase as more of the asymptomatic, undiagnosed patient population become newly diagnosed and aware of their status; however, as treatment is initiated with improved antiviral regimens, the overall prevalence of hepatitis C and more importantly, the complications associated with HCV, will decrease.

CLINICAL MANIFESTATIONS

The acute phase of hepatitis C occurs within days to 6 months after being exposed to HCV. Most patients with acute hepatitis C are asymptomatic; however, some may present with complaints such as jaundice, dark urine, pale stools, right upper quadrant abdominal pain, nausea, fever, anorexia, and fatigue. Routine laboratory values at this time may show markedly elevated serum aminotransferase levels.[12] This acute viral infection will spontaneously clear in 15% to 20% of patients; however, chronic infection will develop in up to 85%.[2,4,10]

Patients who have chronic hepatitis C disease are also largely asymptomatic, however, may complain of nonspecific symptoms such as fatigue, nausea, and myalgia. Serum aminotransferase levels in the chronic phase can vary, and there is virtually no correlation between liver transaminases and the degree of liver disease.[2,4,10] Although chronic hepatitis C disease is typically slow to progress, it can naturally evolve into liver fibrosis, cirrhosis, and HCC.

In addition to the aforementioned generalized complaints, patients with cirrhosis may present with signs of decompensated liver disease such as bilateral lower extremity edema, jaundice, ascites, and asterixis. Laboratory values can vary with cirrhosis and end-stage liver disease, however, may reveal thrombocytopenia, abnormal clotting factors, elevated liver function values (aminotransferases, alkaline phosphatase, γ-glutamyl transpeptidase, bilirubin), and elevated serum creatinine levels.[4,10] Additionally, HCV-related cirrhosis is the most common reason for liver transplantation in the United States.

Patients with HCC may also present with B symptoms, complaining of generalized fatigue, malaise, unexplained weight loss, and anorexia. Alpha-fetoprotein levels are typically elevated in patients with HCC and imaging of the liver via ultrasound scan or MRI will find liver lesions or masses.

Of note, although most patients with chronic hepatitis C disease are asymptomatic, patients can commonly have varying degrees of extrahepatic manifestations, affecting numerous organ/body systems[6,13] including:

- Hematologic (cryoglobulinemia, lymphoma, aplastic anemia)
- Dermatologic (lichen planus, porphyria cutanea tarda)
- Musculoskeletal (myalgias, arthralgias, arthritis, peripheral neuropathy)
- Endocrine (insulin resistance and diabetes, hypothyroidism)
- Autoimmune (thyroiditis, immune thrombocytopenia)
- Renal (glomerulonephritis, nephrotic syndrome)
- Neuropsychiatric (depression, neurocognitive disorders)
- Ocular (corneal ulcers, uveitis)
- Vascular (necrotizing vasculitis)

DIAGNOSTIC AND BASELINE TESTING

Screening for hepatitis C disease is typically performed with a serum HCV antibody test (anti-HCV). Infection with HCV can be detected by anti-HCV 4 to 10 weeks after exposure. For those patients with a reactive HCV antibody test result or suspected acute infection (ie, a history of exposure within the last 6 months), a hepatitis C quantitative viral load by polymerase chain reaction (PCR) is performed. The HCV viral load indicates the amount of hepatitis C virus that is actively replicating and circulating in the bloodstream (ie, viremia), and can detect HCV infection as early as 2 to 3 weeks after exposure (Table 1).[6,10]

Once HCV positivity is confirmed, additional baseline laboratory tests should be ordered in anticipation of creating a treatment plan, such as HCV genotype and subtype,

Table 1		
Interpretation of hepatitis C virus screening results		
HCV Antibody	**HCV Viral Load by PCR**	**Interpretation**
−	−	The patient does not have active HCV infection
−	+	• The patient has active HCV infection ○ Possible recent exposure within the past 6 mo ○ Possible false-negative anti-HCV
+	−	• The patient does not have active HCV infection ○ Possible past exposure and subsequent HCV clearance ○ Possible false-positive anti-HCV (cross-reactivity)
+	+	The patient has active HCV infection

α-fetoprotein, international normalized ratio, HIV screen with a fourth-generation antigen/antibody combination (eg, HIV-1/2 immunoassay), hepatitis A antibody, hepatitis B antigen, hepatitis B antibody quantitative, complete blood cell count, renal function panel with calculated glomerular filtration rate, hepatic function panel, thyroid stimulating hormone, and pregnancy test (if applicable). Additionally, FibroSure should also be considered for baseline laboratory testing in preparation for treatment planning (see details in staging below).

If genotype 1a, further baseline testing for evaluation of the presence of certain preexisting resistance-associated variants (RAV) should also be considered for baseline laboratory testing.[6,14] Commercial laboratory tests typically offer additional options including reflex testing for genotype after a confirmatory HCV PCR and, if genotype 1a, a reflexive genotype 1a NS5A RAV test.

Similar to HIV and hepatitis B virus, HCV has the potential to develop mutations and subsequent resistance patterns, as these viruses all have rapid viral replication rates and are highly error prone because of an RNA-dependent RNA polymerase, which lacks a proofreading function, ultimately resulting in genetically distinct, but closely related, viral variants or quasispecies. These quasispecies may have mutations that confer resistance to anti-HCV regimens; however, this seems to depend on the specific combination of direct-acting antivirals (namely, regimens that include an NS5A inhibitor) and the HCV genotype (primarily with genotype 1a and genotype 3 infections). In fact, it has been cited that 10% to15% of HCV-positive patients with genotype 1 who have not been previously treated with NS5A inhibitors will have detectable NS5A RAVs before treatment. In the future, providers may also consider additional baseline testing with not only HCV genotype and subtype assays, but also with HCV phenotype assays.[6,14] Generally speaking, genotypic assays find specific viral mutations, which may be associated with decreased susceptibilities to antiviral drugs. Phenotypic assays, however, show how the virus with said mutations behaves in the presence of antiviral drugs.

DISEASE STAGING

In addition to determining the HCV genotype, staging is equally important when considering a treatment plan for the hepatitis C–positive patient. Staging directly reflects the progression of hepatitis C disease, which is based on the degree of fibrosis of the hepatocytes (a scarring process secondary to the chronic inflammatory state). The staging process ultimately guides the decisions for treatment based on the urgency to treat, as those who have progressed into cirrhosis are of highest risk for progressive liver disease, extrahepatic complications, liver failure, and HCC and are, therefore, the most urgent to treat.[6]

The gold standard for staging is a liver biopsy with histopathology analysis. There are multiple systems used to define the degree of hepatic fibrosis; however METAVIR is one of the most commonly used. The METAVIR system uses 2 separate scores, one for the grade of necroinflammation or activity (A) and another for the stage of fibrosis (F), as described in Table 2.

Although considered the gold standard for staging, most providers do not obtain liver biopsies for many reasons, including the cost and invasive nature of the procedure (with the consideration of recovery time), possible complications, and sampling error/variability. Providers are now often opting for an alternative, less-invasive, and more cost-efficient method of staging via imaging (with liver ultrasound scan, liver MRI, or ultrasound-based transient elastography/FibroScan [Echosens, Paris, France]) or via laboratory evaluation (with FibroSure or the aspartate aminotransferase/platelet ratio index [APRI]).

Table 2	
The METAVIR system	
Necroinflammation or Activity	Stage of Fibrosis
A0 = no activity	F0 = no fibrosis
A1 = minimal activity	F1 = portal fibrosis
A2 = moderate activity	F2 = bridging fibrosis with few septa
A3 = severe activity	F3 = bridging fibrosis with many septa
	F4 = cirrhosis

Ultrasound-based transient elastography, or FibroScan, is an ultrasound-guided examination of the liver that measures liver stiffness (liver elasticity and viscosity) as mechanical excitation is applied to the liver via shear waves or compression. The flexibility of the liver tissue is then measured and correlated to the degree of liver fibrosis. Transient elastography has a sensitivity of 70% and a specificity of 84% for diagnosing significant hepatic fibrosis (F2-3 using the METAVIR staging system) and a sensitivity of 87% and a specificity of 91% for diagnosing cirrhosis.[15] Although transient elastography is highly accurate in determining the stage of fibrosis, the cost and availability of this procedure remain obstacles.

FibroSure is a blood test offered commercially that uses 6 biochemical markers (α2-macroglobulin, haptoglobin, apolipoprotein A1, total bilirubin, γ-glutamyl transpeptidase, and alanine aminotransferase) combined with a patient's age and sex into an algorithm, which, in turn, generates a measure of fibrosis and necroinflammatory activity in the liver, corresponding to the METAVIR scoring system mentioned above.[16] FibroSure has a sensitivity of 60% to 75% and a specificity of 80% to 90% for predicting significant hepatic fibrosis.[17,18] Although the FibroSure test is less invasive and more cost efficient than a liver biopsy, it has its limitations. Several medical conditions (eg, Gilbert disease, acute hepatitis, extrahepatic cholestasis, or transplant patients) and certain medications (eg, atazanavir) can affect 1 or more of the 6 biochemical markers, thereby causing misinterpretation and incorrect assignment of the scores of liver fibrosis and necroinflammatory activity.[16]

The APRI is a score that can be quickly calculated from routine laboratory values and can help predict significant hepatic fibrosis. An APRI score greater than 1.0 has a sensitivity of 76% and specificity of 72% for predicting cirrhosis, and an APRI score greater than 0.7 has a sensitivity of 77% and specificity of 72% for predicting significant hepatic fibrosis (F2-3 using the METAVIR staging system).[17,19] Although the APRI is quick and cost effective, it is not sensitive enough to independently rule out significant liver disease and is typically used in conjunction with other modalities.

In the SAFE (Sequential Algorithm for Fibrosis Evaluation) biopsy study,[20] for example, researchers sought to use a combination of APRI and FibroSure to predict the level of fibrosis followed by liver biopsies in a subset of cases, with the goal of reducing the number of liver biopsies needed. The algorithm proved to guarantee greater than 90% diagnostic accuracy (compared with liver histology, the gold standard) and had less than 2% underestimation in the stage of liver disease. Additionally, the discordant cases (SAFE biopsy vs liver biopsy results) were further evaluated with FibroScan, which confirmed results of the SAFE biopsy in 81%.[20]

ASSESSING TREATMENT HISTORY

Another important part of the patient history to obtain before determining an appropriate treatment regimen is their prior HCV treatment history. Treatment-naïve patients have never had treatment for HCV. Patients treated previously with PEGylated interferon (with or without ribavirin) can be categorized as prior relapsers, partial responders, or null responders. Patients could have also been treated previously and not responded to protease-inhibitor regimens (boceprevir, simeprevir, or telaprevir) or sofosbuvir-based regimens.[6]

TREATMENT BASICS

Once the genotype, staging, and treatment history have been determined, a treatment plan can be formulated for the patient with chronic hepatitis C. The goal of therapy is to achieve an SVR, which is defined as having no detectable virus in the bloodstream (via quantitative HCV RNA PCR) at 12 to 24 weeks after completion of antiviral therapy. Once SVR is achieved, the patient is considered clinically cured, which ultimately reduces HCV-related morbidity (such as hepatic decompensation and the development of hepatocellular carcinoma) and mortality.

Historically, the treatment of chronic hepatitis C consisted of combination therapy with PEGylated interferon injections plus oral ribavirin, a regimen that was both difficult to tolerate and poorly efficacious, with varying SVR rates up to 55% (46% for genotype 1 and 82% for genotype 2/3).[2] Adverse effects such as flulike symptoms, fatigue, depression, and alopecia were commonly reported as moderate to severe in intensity, and the sometimes profound bone marrow suppression (anemia, neutropenia, and thrombocytopenia) required frequent follow-up visits for close laboratory monitoring and concomitant growth factors (such as Procrit or Neupogen) and occasionally warranted hospital admission for blood product support. Further complicating HCV treatment, PEGylated interferon plus ribavirin usually required prolonged durations, depending on the genotype (up to 48 weeks for genotype 1). Because of the difficulty of this treatment regimen, only those patients with advanced liver disease (compensated cirrhosis) or those at high risk for complications were treated. Others, who were at lower risk for progression of liver disease and subsequent complications, were treated expectantly and observed clinically in hopes of improved treatment regimens in the future.

With the introduction of direct-acting antivirals (DAAs), several treatment regimens are available that are all oral and have markedly improved side-effect profiles, higher rates of SVR, and shorter durations of therapy (Tables 3 and 4). DAA regimens are being developed rapidly; therefore, recommendations also change rapidly. By the time this article is published, there will be several new single-tablet regimens that are pan-genotypic and have SVRs approaching 100% for all genotypes. The joint guidelines published by AASLD and IDSA[6] will continue to be a useful reference for up-to-date recommended regimens for the treatment of chronic hepatitis C.

Generally speaking, with regard to patient selection for hepatitis C therapy, anyone who is chronically infected with hepatitis C should be treated, except for those patients with short life expectancies who would not benefit from HCV treatment. If resources are limited, however, priority for treatment (per joint AASLD/IDSA guidelines[6]) should be given to:

- Patients with advanced liver disease (F3-4 on the METAVIR staging system)
- Patients with severe extrahepatic manifestations of HCV
- Transplant recipients
- Patients with HIV or hepatitis B co-infection
- Patients with concomitant liver disease
- Patients with diabetes mellitus
- Patients at high risk of transmitting HCV (intravenous drug users, HIV-positive men who have sex with men, incarcerated patients, and patients on hemodialysis)

Table 3
Pharmacology of direct-acting antivirals

Classes of DAAs	Mechanism of Action	Common Side Effects
NS3/4A protease inhibitors	Inhibit NS3/4A serine protease	
Grazoprevir	(Posttranslational processing and HCV replication)	
Paritaprevir		
Simeprevir		Rash, photosensitivity, hyperbilirubinemia
NS5A inhibitors	Inhibit NS5A protein	
Daclatasvir	(HCV replication and assembly)	Headache, fatigue, nausea
Elbasvir		
Ledipasvir		
Ombitasvir		
Velpatasvir		
NS5B RNA-dependant RNA polymerase inhibitors	Inhibit NS5B polymerase (posttranslational processing and HCV replication)	
NPI: Sofosbuvir	Nucleoside/nucleotide analogue (NPI)	Headache, fatigue, nausea, insomnia, anemia
NNPI: Dasabuvir	Non-nucleoside analogue (NNPI)	
Fixed-dose combinations		
Elbasvir-grazoprevir		Headache, fatigue, nausea
Ledipasvir-sofosbuvir		Headache, fatigue, nausea, insomnia
Ombitasvir-paritaprevir-ritonavir ± dasabuvir		Nausea, pruritus, insomnia, diarrhea, asthenia
Sofosbuvir-velpatasvir		Headache, fatigue, nausea, nasopharyngitis, insomnia

Abbreviations: NPI, Nucleot(s)ide polymerase inhibitor; NNPI, Nonnucleoside polymerase inhibitor.

Possible drug-drug interactions must be carefully considered when choosing a potential antiviral regimen for an HCV-positive patient, as many of the DAAs are metabolized by the cytochrome P450 system. Because of the short duration of these DAA regimens, however, (12–24 weeks of therapy), clinicians may consider choosing alternative options for concomitant medications.

DAA regimens can be costly, running upwards of $100,000 for a treatment course (12–24 weeks of therapy); however, many pharmaceutical companies offer patient assistance programs and copayment coupons to help make the regimen more affordable for HCV-positive patients.

TREATING HEPATITIS C IN SPECIAL POPULATIONS

Treatment regimens may vary for a few select special populations, including patients with HIV/hepatitis C co-infection and those with chronic kidney disease.

Table 4
Hepatitis C virus treatment regimens

	Duration	Additional Info
Genotype 1a Treatment-Naïve Patients Without Cirrhosis		
Recommended Regimen		
Daily fixed-dose combination of elbasvir (50 mg)/grazoprevir (100 mg)	12 wk	NO baseline NS5A RAVs for elbasvir are detected
Daily fixed-dose combination of ledipasvir (90 mg)/sofosbuvir (400 mg)	12 wk	
Daily fixed-dose combination of paritaprevir (150 mg)/ritonavir (100 mg)/ombitasvir (25 mg) plus twice-daily dosed dasabuvir (250 mg) with weight-based ribavirin	12 wk	
Daily simeprevir (150 mg) plus sofosbuvir (400 mg)	12 wk	
Daily fixed-dose combination of sofosbuvir (400 mg)/velpatasvir (100 mg)	12 wk	
Daily daclatasvir (60 mg*) plus sofosbuvir (400 mg)	12 wk	
Alternative Regimen		
Daily fixed-dose combination of elbasvir (50 mg)/grazoprevir (100 mg) with weight-based ribavirin	16 wk	Baseline NS5A RAVs for elbasvir ARE detected
Genotype 1a Treatment-Naïve Patients with Compensated Cirrhosis		
Recommended Regimen		
Daily fixed-dose combination of elbasvir (50 mg)/grazoprevir (100 mg)	12 wk	NO baseline NS5A RAVs for elbasvir are detected
Daily fixed-dose combination of ledipasvir (90 mg)/sofosbuvir (400 mg)	12 wk	
Daily fixed-dose combination of sofosbuvir (400 mg)/velpatasvir (100 mg)	12 wk	
Alternative Regimen		
Daily fixed-dose combination of paritaprevir (150 mg)/ritonavir (100 mg)/ombitasvir (25 mg) plus twice-daily dosed dasabuvir (250 mg) with weight-based ribavirin	24 wk	
Daily simeprevir (150 mg) plus sofosbuvir (400 mg) with or without weight-based ribavirin	24 wk	NO Q80K polymorphism is detected
Daily daclatasvir (60 mg*) plus sofosbuvir (400 mg) with or without weight-based ribavirin	24 wk	
Daily fixed-dose combination of elbasvir (50 mg)/grazoprevir (100 mg) with weight-based ribavirin	16 wk	Baseline NS5A RAVs for elbasvir ARE detected
Genotype 1b Treatment-Naïve Patients Without Cirrhosis		
Recommended Regimen		
Daily fixed-dose combination of elbasvir (50 mg)/grazoprevir (100 mg)	12 wk	

(continued on next page)

Table 4 (*continued*)	Duration	Additional Info
Daily fixed-dose combination of ledipasvir (90 mg)/sofosbuvir (400 mg)	12 wk	
Daily fixed-dose combination of paritaprevir (150 mg)/ritonavir (100 mg)/ombitasvir (25 mg) plus twice-daily dosed dasabuvir (250 mg)	12 wk	
Daily simeprevir (150 mg) plus sofosbuvir (400 mg)	12 wk	
Daily fixed-dose combination of sofosbuvir (400 mg)/velpatasvir (100 mg)	12 wk	
Daily daclatasvir (60 mg*) plus sofosbuvir (400 mg)	12 wk	
Genotype 1b Treatment-Naïve Patients with Compensated Cirrhosis		
Recommended Regimen		
Daily fixed-dose combination of elbasvir (50 mg)/grazoprevir (100 mg)	12 wk	
Daily fixed-dose combination of ledipasvir (90 mg)/sofosbuvir (400 mg)	12 wk	
Daily fixed-dose combination of paritaprevir (150 mg)/ritonavir (100 mg)/ombitasvir (25 mg) plus twice-daily dosed dasabuvir (250 mg)	12 wk	
Daily fixed-dose combination of sofosbuvir (400 mg)/velpatasvir (100 mg)	12 wk	
Alternative Regimen		
Daily daclatasvir (60 mg*) plus sofosbuvir (400 mg) with or without weight-based ribavirin	24 wk	
Daily simeprevir (150 mg) plus sofosbuvir (400 mg) with or without weight-based ribavirin	24 wk	
Genotype 2 Treatment-Naïve Patients Without Cirrhosis		
Recommended Regimen		
Daily fixed-dose combination of sofosbuvir (400 mg)/velpatasvir (100 mg)	12 wk	
Alternative Regimen		
Daily daclatasvir (60 mg*) plus sofosbuvir (400 mg)	12 wk	
Genotype 2 Treatment-Naïve Patients with Compensated Cirrhosis		
Recommended Regimen		
Daily fixed-dose combination of sofosbuvir (400 mg)/velpatasvir (100 mg)	12 wk	
Alternative Regimen		
Daily daclatasvir (60 mg*) plus sofosbuvir (400 mg)	16–24 wk	

(*continued on next page*)

Table 4
(continued)

	Duration	Additional Info
Genotype 3 Treatment-Naïve Patients Without Cirrhosis		
Recommended Regimen		
Daily daclatasvir (60 mg*) plus sofosbuvir (400 mg)	12 wk	
Daily fixed-dose combination of sofosbuvir (400 mg)/velpatasvir (100 mg)	12 wk	
Genotype 3 Treatment-Naïve Patients with Compensated Cirrhosis		
Recommended Regimen		
Daily fixed-dose combination of sofosbuvir (400 mg)/velpatasvir (100 mg)	12 wk	
Daily daclatasvir (60 mg*) plus sofosbuvir (400 mg) with or without weight-based ribavirin	24 wk	RAV testing for Y93H is recommended for cirrhotic patients. If present, add ribavirin
Genotype 4 Treatment-Naïve Patients Without Cirrhosis		
Recommended Regimen		
Daily fixed-dose combination of paritaprevir (150 mg)/ritonavir (100 mg)/ombitasvir (25 mg) and weight-based ribavirin	12 wk	
Daily fixed-dose combination of sofosbuvir (400 mg)/velpatasvir (100 mg)	12 wk	
Daily fixed-dose combination of elbasvir (50 mg)/grazoprevir (100 mg)	12 wk	
Daily fixed-dose combination of ledipasvir (90 mg)/sofosbuvir (400 mg)	12 wk	
Genotype 4 Treatment-Naïve Patients with Compensated Cirrhosis		
Recommended Regimen		
Daily fixed-dose combination of paritaprevir (150 mg)/ritonavir (100 mg)/ombitasvir (25 mg) and weight-based ribavirin	12 wk	
Daily fixed-dose combination of sofosbuvir (400 mg)/velpatasvir (100 mg)	12 wk	
Daily fixed-dose combination of elbasvir (50 mg)/grazoprevir (100 mg)	12 wk	
Daily fixed-dose combination of ledipasvir (90 mg)/sofosbuvir (400 mg)	12 wk	
Genotype 5/6 Treatment-Naïve Patients with and Without Cirrhosis		
Recommended Regimen		
Daily fixed-dose combination of sofosbuvir (400 mg)/velpatasvir (100 mg)	12 wk	
Daily fixed-dose combination of ledipasvir (90 mg)/sofosbuvir (400 mg)	12 wk	

* Dose may need to be adjusted if given concomitantly with P450 3A/4 inducers or inhibitors.

It is well known that patients co-infected with HCV and HIV have an accelerated rate of disease progression and are, therefore, considered to be high priority to treat. Treatment in this special population is typically undertaken by or in consultation with an expert (infectious diseases, HIV specialist, or hepatology) when deciding on an HCV treatment regimen, as there are potentially severe drug-drug interactions between the HIV antivirals and the HCV antivirals. HIV regimens can be adjusted before starting the preferred hepatitis C therapy; however, HIV treatment interruptions to treat hepatitis C are not recommended.[6]

In patients with chronic kidney disease, both the HCV genotype and the stage of kidney disease are used in treatment planning, as some regimens have limitations in patients with severe renal impairment or end-stage renal disease.

OCCUPATIONAL EXPOSURE CONSIDERATIONS

The rate of transmission of HCV via occupational exposure is up to 3%.[4,21] There are currently no recommendations for postexposure prophylaxis (PEP) after an occupational exposure to a source patient with HCV, and these patients are typically followed up with serial laboratory work (typically at baseline and at 6 weeks, 3 months, and 6 months from the date of exposure) with an HCV antibody or quantitative HCV viral load by PCR. The goal for follow-up is the early detection and treatment of any positive seroconversion; however, the traditional expectant management style of postexposure protocol for HCV may be soon reconsidered with the advent of DAA regimens. As noted above, the present-day regimens used to treat chronic HCV are generally well tolerated and have dosing frequencies that allow for excellent compliance, similar to the HIV PEP regimens taken by patients after an exposure to a source patient that is HIV positive. These HIV PEP regimens allow for a significant decrease in the rate of transmission of HIV, protecting those patients with occupational exposures. Admittedly, up to 20% of those patients that have seroconversion to HCV positive status after an exposure may still have spontaneous clearance of the acute infection; however, treatment during this acute phase is correlated with excellent rates of SVR.[12] The cost of hepatitis C therapy is the only drawback; however, looking forward, providers may be reconsidering treating high-risk occupational exposures (those with known HCV-positive sources) for HCV empirically.

THE FUTURE OF HEPATITIS C VIRUS: A BEGINNING TO AN END

The future is bright for those patients living with chronic hepatitis C, as there are now numerous regimens commercially available with excellent tolerability and efficacy. As providers in all areas of medicine become more familiar with the HCV screening guidelines and new treatment regimens, there is hope for an overall increase in those clinically cured of their HCV disease and a subsequent marked decrease in HCV-related morbidity and mortality. Notably, the eradication of hepatitis C globally has been mentioned recently by experts as a truly attainable goal.

REFERENCES

1. Mandell GL, Bennett JE, Dolin R. Principles and practice of infectious diseases. Philadelphia: The Curtis Center; 2005.
2. Schlossberg David, editor. Clinical infectious disease. New York: Cambridge University Press; 2008.
3. Chevaliez S, Pawlotsky JM. HCV genome and life cycle. In: Hepatitis C viruses: genomes and molecular biology. Norfolk (United Kingdom): 2006. Chapter 1.

Available at: Error! Hyperlink reference not valid.www.ncbi.nlm.nih.gov/books/NBK1630/. Accessed June 23, 2016.

4. Hepatitis C. Available at: http://emedicine.medscape.com/article/177792-overview#a5. Accessed July 3, 2016.

5. Messina JP, Humphreys I, Flaxman A, et al. Global distribution and prevalence of hepatitis C virus genotypes. Hepatology 2015;61:77–87.

6. AASLD/IDSA. Recommendations for testing, managing and treating Hepatitis C. Available at: http://www.hcvguidelines.org. 2015. Accessed July 7, 2016.

7. Kim CW, Chang KM. Hepatitis C virus: virology and life cycle. Clin Mol Hepatol 2013;19(1):17–25.

8. Neumann AU, Lam NP, Dahari H, et al. Hepatitis C viral dynamics in vivo and the antiviral efficacy of interferon-alpha therapy. Science 1998;282(5386):103–7.

9. Moradpour D, Penin F. Hepatitis C virus proteins: from structure to function. Curr Top Microbiol Immunol 2013;369:113–42.

10. Viral Hepatitis- Hepatitis C Information. Available at: http://www.cdc.gov/hepatitis/hcv/hcvfaq.htm. Accessed July 21, 2016.

11. Management of Hepatitis C. Available at: http://consensus.nih.gov/1997/1997HepatitisC105html.htm. 1997. Accessed June 8, 2016.

12. Maheshwari A, Ray S, Thuluvath PJ. Acute Hepatitis C. Lancet 2008;372(9635):321–32.

13. Cacoub P, Renou C, Rosenthal E, et al. Extrahepatic manifestations associated with hepatitis C virus infection. A prospective multicenter study of 321 patients. The GERMIVIC. Medicine (Baltimore) 2000;79(1):47–56.

14. Kieffer TL, Kwong AD, Picchio GR. Viral resistance to specifically targeted antiviral therapies for hepatitis C (STAT-Cs). J Antimicrob Chemother 2010;65:202–12.

15. Talwalkar JA, Kurtz DM, Schoenleber SJ, et al. Ultrasound-based transient elastography for the detection of hepatic fibrosis: systematic review and meta-analysis. Clin Gastroenterol Hepatol 2007;5(10):1214.

16. HCV Fibrosure™. Available at: http://www.hemophilia.co.il/documents/Fibrotest.pdf. Accessed July 9, 2016.

17. Chou R, Wasson N. Blood tests to diagnose fibrosis or cirrhosis in patients with chronic hepatitis C virus infection: a systematic review. Ann Intern Med 2013;158:807–20.

18. Halfon P, Bourliere M, Deydier R, et al. TI Independent prospective multicenter validation of biochemical markers (fibrotest-actitest) for the prediction of liver fibrosis and activity in patients with chronic hepatitis C: the fibropaca study. Am J Gastroenterol 2006;101(3):547–55.

19. Lin ZH, Xin YN, Dong QJ, et al. Performance of the aspartate aminotransferase-to-platelet ratio index for the staging of hepatitis C-related fibrosis: an updated meta-analysis. Hepatology 2011;53:726–36.

20. Sebastiani G, Halfon P, Castera L, et al. SAFE biopsy: a validated method for large-scale staging of liver fibrosis in chronic hepatitis C. Hepatology 2009;49(6):1821–7.

21. U.S. Public Health Service. Updated U.S. Public Health Service Guidelines for the Management of Occupational Exposures to HBV, HCV, and HIV and Recommendations for Postexposure Prophylaxis. MMWR Recomm Rep 2001;50:1–42.

Update on Human Immunodeficiency Virus

Michelle Touw, PA-C, MMS

KEYWORDS

- Human immunodeficiency virus (HIV) • HIV care continuum
- Opportunistic infection (OI) • Antiretroviral therapy (ART)
- Acute retroviral syndrome (ARS) • Pre-exposure prophylaxis (PrEP)

KEY POINTS

- Only 83% of people living with human immunodeficiency virus (HIV) in the United States are aware of their HIV infection, and only 25% of people living with HIV have full viral suppression.
- HIV acquisition risk can be reduced by identifying at-risk individuals and educating them on safe sex practices including condom use, identifying and treating sexually transmitted infections, pre-exposure prophylaxis, and in certain groups, male circumcision.
- Health care providers should consider HIV and opportunistic infections in the differential diagnosis of acutely ill patients.
- Antiretroviral therapy is very effective at treating HIV, and patients who achieve full viral suppression have improved long-term survival, and reduced risk for cardiac, renal, and neoplastic diseases.

INTRODUCTION

Human immunodeficiency virus (HIV) disease continues to be a major health issue, and recent public health efforts are focused on identifying at-risk and newly infected individuals. In the United States, African American men who have sex with men (MSM) have the highest risk for acquiring HIV.[1] Early treatment with the newer and more tolerable antiretroviral drugs reduces the rate of opportunistic infections (OI) and aims to reduce the spread of HIV infections.[2] Health care providers should screen patients at risk for HIV acquisition and offer testing.[3] OIs still occur in undiagnosed and untreated patients, and HIV disease and OIs should be considered in the differential diagnosis of acutely ill patients. Newer medications are much more tolerable than in the past, and most patients can take medications once daily or even single-tablet regimens (STR).

Disclosure Statement: The author has nothing to disclose.
Division of Infectious Diseases, Department of Internal Medicine, Eastern Virginia Medical School, 825 Fairfax Avenue, Norfolk, VA 23507, USA
E-mail address: touwm@evms.edu

Physician Assist Clin 2 (2017) 327–343
http://dx.doi.org/10.1016/j.cpha.2016.12.013
2405-7991/17/© 2017 Elsevier Inc. All rights reserved.

physicianassistant.theclinics.com

EPIDEMIOLOGY

Despite excellent advances in prevention and treatment, the HIV epidemic continues with greater than 35 million people living with HIV (PLWHIV) worldwide. Sub-Saharan Africa remains most severely affected, with 25 million people, nearly 1 in every 20 adults, living with HIV.[4] Outside of Africa, most new infections are in key populations with specific risk factors.

More than 1.2 million people in the United States are living with HIV infection, and almost 1 in 8 (12.8%) are unaware of their infection. Gay, bisexual, and other MSM of all races and ethnicities remain the most profoundly affected by HIV.[1] Significant racial disparities exist with 40% of diagnoses in 2014 identified in African American men, whereas African American men made up 12% of the total US population (Fig. 1, Table 1). Rates of acquired immunodeficiency syndrome (AIDS) diagnosis and deaths due to AIDS also disproportionately affect African Americans, with the death rate nearly 4 times higher than any other ethnic group (Fig. 2).

Recent public health efforts have focused on treatment as prevention (TasP) and increasing the identification and treatment of newly infected individuals, because the overall viremia in these patients is much higher, which may increase the risk of transmission. HIV surveillance in the United States shows that only 30% of PLWHIV have VL suppression[1] (Fig. 3). The HIV care continuum goals are to diagnose at-risk patients, link patients to care, prescribe antiretroviral therapy (ART), and achieve full viral suppression.

VIRAL CHARACTERISTICS

HIV is an enveloped RNA lentivirus with an icosahedral structure and external protein spikes formed by GP 120 and GP 41 proteins. HIV infects CD4 cells by binding to the GP 120 protein and CCR5 or X4 receptors, causing a conformational change in the virus that allows it to enter into the cytoplasm of host cells. HIV uses the enzyme reverse

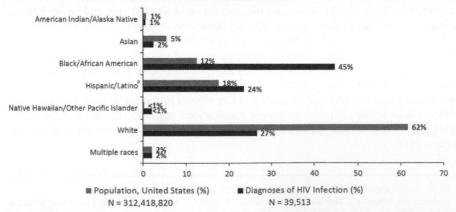

Fig. 1. Diagnoses of HIV infection population and race in men. *Note*: Data include persons with a diagnosis of HIV infection regardless of stage of disease at diagnosis. Data for the year 2015 are preliminary and based on 6 months reporting delay. [a] Hispanics/Latinos can be of any race. (*From* CDC Resource Library. HIV Surveillance by Race/Ethnicity (through 2015). Available at: http://www.cdc.gov/hiv/library/slidesets/index.html. Accessed September 2, 2016.)

Table 1
Diagnoses of human immunodeficiency virus infection by population and race

Race/Ethnicity	No.	Rate
American Indian/Alaska Native	55	2.3
Asian[a]	55	0.3
Black/African American	6888	17.4
Hispanic/Latino[b]	2525	4.6
Native Hawaiian/Other Pacific Islander	7	1.3
White	4722	2.4
Multiple races	867	13.6
Total	*15,119*	*4.7*

Note: Data include persons with a diagnosis of HIV infection regardless of stage of disease at diagnosis. Deaths of persons with diagnosed HIV may be due to any cause.
    [a] Includes Asian/Pacific Islander legacy cases.
    [b] Hispanics/Latinos can be of any race.
    From CDC Resource Library. HIV Surveillance by Race/Ethnicity (through 2015). Available at: http://www.cdc.gov/hiv/library/slidesets/index.html. Accessed September 2, 2016.

transcriptase to convert viral RNA to proviral DNA, which then uses the integrase enzyme to move from the cytoplasm to the nucleus of the CD4 cell.[5] CD4 cell activation is a key step in HIV disease pathogenesis. Activated CD4 cells trigger replication of viral RNA and proteins, allowing new virions to be formed and bud from the surface of infected CD4 cells and then spread to other cells[5] (see "The HIV Life Cycle" infographic at: https://aidsinfo.nih.gov/education-materials/fact-sheets/19/73/the-hiv-life-cycle).

HIV originated from primate viruses circulating among different groups in Africa. Both HIV-1 and HIV-2 have multiple groups and subtypes that may account for the

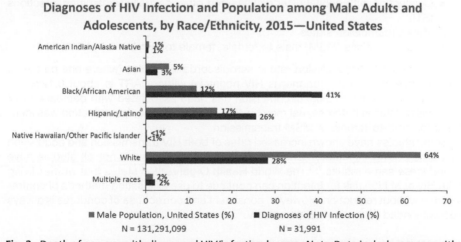

Diagnoses of HIV Infection and Population among Male Adults and Adolescents, by Race/Ethnicity, 2015—United States

■ Male Population, United States (%)   ■ Diagnoses of HIV Infection (%)
N = 131,291,099   N = 31,991

Fig. 2. Death of persons with diagnosed HIV/infection by race. *Note*: Data include persons with a diagnosis of HIV infection regardless of stage of disease at diagnosis. Data for the year 2015 are preliminary and based on 6 months reporting delay. [a] Hispanics/Latinos can be of any race. (*From* CDC resource library. HIV surveillance by race/ethnicity (through 2015). Available at: http://www.cdc.gov/hiv/library/slidesets/index.html. Accessed September 2, 2016.)

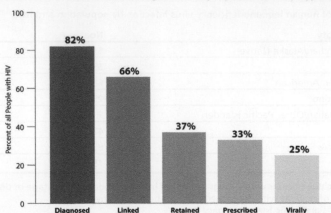

Fig. 3. Viral suppression in the United States. (*From* CDC vital signs. HIV stages of care. CDC fact sheet. Available at: http://www.cdc.gov/nchhstp/newsroom/2014/hiv-stages-of-care. html. Accessed September 2, 2016.)

variability in disease progression. HIV-1 is the most common form of the virus worldwide and is predominately in the United States and Europe. HIV-2 originated from a primate more common to West Africa and is associated with lower VLs and slower declines in CD4 count.[5]

HUMAN IMMUNODEFICIENCY VIRUS TRANSMISSION

Factors that affect the efficiency of HIV transmission include the following:

- HIV viral load (VL)
- Coinfection with genital ulcer disease and other sexually transmitted infections (STI)
- Male circumcision status
- Sexual practices (MSM, male to female, female to male)

The overall HIV transmission rate in serodiscordant couples (where one partner is HIV positive and another partner is HIV negative) without ART is about 0.12% per act.[5] In Africa, male medical circumcision has been associated with decreased HIV acquisition rates in heterosexual men by 40% to 60%, but no risk reduction was identified for male-to-female or MSM transmission.[6]

Some studies have shown increased rates of both HIV transmission and acquisition in women using injectable hormonal contraception; however, not all studies have found these same results.[7,8] The World Health Organization states that women living with HIV or at high risk for infection can continue to use all existing methods of contraception without restriction. However, consistent and correct use of condoms is always recommended to prevent spread of HIV.[7]

HUMAN IMMUNODEFICIENCY VIRUS TESTING

The Centers for Disease Control and Prevention (CDC) recommends that all individuals 13 to 64 years old have a screening test for HIV at least once and that patients should be informed that an HIV test will be performed unless the patient opts out.

More frequent HIV testing should be performed in certain groups, including patients being treated for tuberculosis or with signs or symptoms of HIV infection.[9] Routine screening every 3 to 6 months or after a high-risk exposure is recommended for patients with risk factors, such as[3]:

- MSM
- Anonymous sexual contacts
- A recent positive test for another STI
- Injection drug use
- Contact with a known HIV-positive partner

The fourth-generation HIV test screens for HIV-1 and HIV-2 antibody (AB) as well as p24 antigen, which is present in the blood as early as 3 weeks after infection with HIV.[9] This test reduces the rate of false negative tests significantly and may identify patients during acute retroviral syndrome (ARS).

HUMAN IMMUNODEFICIENCY VIRUS PREVENTION

Epidemiologically, the MSM population has the overall highest risk of HIV acquisition due to prevalence of HIV and sexual practices in this population. Recent studies have focused on methods to reduce the infection rate in high-risk groups including both pre-exposure prophylaxis (PrEP) and postexposure prophylaxis (PEP) for sexual exposure to HIV.[10] A recent European trial[11] has shown up to 86% reduced risk in MSM who took PrEP on demand versus daily use. The regimen recommendations in this study advised subjects to take 1 to 2 tablets of tenofovir/emtricitabine (FTC) 2 to 6 hours before the sex contact and 2 additional doses at 24 and 48 hours after contact. Daily dosing could continue up to 48 hours after the last contact if there were multiple exposure events. Condom use is always recommended to reduce exposure risk for HIV and other STIs. PrEP may also be recommended to reduce the risk of HIV transmission in serodiscordant couples, especially if an HIV-negative woman may be trying to conceive[12] (Table 2).

PEP is a 28-day treatment course given as emergency treatment after high-risk exposure either due to health care–associated exposure or other event. In 2012, CDC released recommendations for use of PEP after a high-risk sexual exposure event, such as condom failure or sexual assault. Medication should be initiated within 72 hours of the event and should be coupled with rapid HIV testing to insure the exposed person is not already HIV positive. The patient should be administered 2 to 3 antiretroviral medications that should be taken for 28 days. Medication choice should be patient specific to avoid drug interactions or adverse events due to underlying conditions. Needle exposure in health care workers is considered a high-risk exposure and is an indication for PEP; however, the relative risk of HIV seroconversion is much lower for HIV than it is for hepatitis C or hepatitis B.[13]

HUMAN IMMUNODEFICIENCY VIRUS CLINICAL STAGES

HIV disease is categorized into the following 3 phases[5]:

- Acute symptomatic infection/acute retroviral syndrome (ARS)
- Latent asymptomatic HIV infection
- Symptomatic disease, including advanced AIDS

HIV disease is also categorized by stages based on CD4 count and VL and clinical signs[14] (Table 3).

	MSM	Heterosexual women and men	Injection drug users
Table 2			
Summary of pre-exposure prophylaxis guidelines			
Detecting substantial risk for HIV infection	HIV-positive sexual partner	HIV-positive sexual partner	HIV-positive injecting partner
	Recent bacterial STI	Recent bacterial STI	Sharing injection equipment
	High number of sex partners	High number of sex partners	Recent drug treatment (but currently injecting)
	History of inconsistent or no condom use	History of inconsistent or no condom use	
	Commercial sex work	Commercial sex work	
		In high-prevalence area or network	
Clinically eligible	Documented negative HIV test result before prescribing PrEP		
	No symptoms/signs of acute HIV infection		
	Normal renal function; no contraindicated medications		
	Documented HBV infection and vaccination status		
Prescription	**Daily, continuing oral doses of TDF-FTC (Truvada; Gilead Sciences); ≤90-d supply**		
Other services	Follow-up visits at least every 3 mo to provide the following: HIV test, medication adherence counseling, behavioral risk-reduction support, side-effect assessment, STI symptom assessment		
	At 3 mo and every 6 mo thereafter, assess renal function		
	Every 6 mo, test for bacterial STIs		
	Do oral/rectal STI testing	Assess pregnancy intent, pregnancy test every 3 mo	Access to clean needles/syringes and drug treatment services

Adapted from Preexposure prophylaxis for the prevention of HIV infection in the United States—2014 clinical practice guideline. p. 11–67. Available at: http://www.cdc.gov/hiv/pdf/guidelines/PrEP guidelines2014.pdf. Accessed September 2, 2016.

Patients with CD4 counts greater than 500 will not generally develop any OIs; however, HIV is a risk factor for cardiovascular disease and non–AIDS–related cancers likely due to systemic inflammation secondary to HIV viremia.[5] Deaths in AIDS patients are only due to AIDS-defining illnesses and related OIs in less than 50% of cases.[15,16]

The presence of an OI at any CD4 count is a diagnosis of AIDS[14] (**Box 1**).

Acute Symptomatic Human Immunodeficiency Virus Infection

Many patients who are recently infected with HIV will present with an ARS 2-4 weeks after exposure with the most common symptoms being

- Fever
- Lymphadenopathy
- Sore throat
- Rash
- Myalgia/arthralgia
- Headache
- Mucocutaneous ulcers

Although these symptoms are not specific to HIV infection, patients with the above symptoms without identification of another source may suggest ARS.[17] Symptoms related to ARS will usually resolve within 2 weeks, and patients rarely return to care once the symptoms resolve. VL testing is still the most reliable method for identifying

Table 3
Centers for Disease Control and Prevention classification by stages

Stage	Laboratory Evidence[a]	Clinical Evidence
Stage 1	Laboratory confirmation of HIV infection *and* CD4+ T-lymphocyte count of ≥500 cells/μL *or* CD4+ T-lymphocyte percentage of ≥29	None required (but no AIDS-defining condition)
Stage 2	Laboratory confirmation of HIV infection *and* CD+ T-lymphocyte count of 200–499 cells/μL *or* CD4+ T-lymphocyte percentage of 14–28	None required (but no AIDS-defining condition)
Stage 3 (AIDS)	Laboratory confirmation of HIV infection *and* CD4+ T-lymphocyte count of <200 cells/μL *or* CD4+ T-lymphocyte percentage of <14[b]	*Or* documentation of an AIDS-defining condition (with laboratory confirmation of HIV infection)[b]
Stage unknown[c]	Laboratory conformation of HIV infection *and* no information on CD4+ T-lymphocyte count *or* percentage	*And* no information on presence of AIDS-defining conditions

[a] The CD4+ T-lymphocyte percentage is the percentage of total lymphocytes. If the CD4+ T-lymphocyte count and percentage do not correspond to the same HIV infection stage, then select the more severe stage.

[b] Documentation of an AIDS-defining condition (Appendix A) supersedes a CD4+ T-lymphocyte count of ≥200 cell/μL and a CD4 T-lymphocyte percentage and total lymphocytes of ≥14. Definitive diagnostic methods for these conditions are available in Appendix C of the 1993 revised HIV classification system and the expanded AIDS case definition (CDC. 1993 Revised Classification System for HIV infection and expanded surveillance case definition for AIDS among adolescents and adults MMWR 1992;41;RR-17) and from the National Notifiable Diseases Surveillance System (Available at: http://www.cdc.gov.epo/dphsi/casedct/case_definitions.htm).

[c] Although cases with no information on CD4+ T-lymphocyte count or percentage or on the presence of AIDS-defining conditions can be classified as stage unknown, every effort should be made to report CD4+ T-lymphocyte counts or percentages and the presence of AIDS-defining conditions at the time of diagnosis. Additional CD4+ T-lymphocyte counts or percentages and any identified AIDS-defining conditions can be reported as recommended (Council of State and Territorial Epidemiologists. Laboratory reporting of clinical test results indicative of HIV infection: new standards for a new era of surveillance and prevention [Position Statement 04-ID-07]; 2004. Available at: http://www.cste.org/ps/2004pdf/04-1D-07-final.pdf.)

From Schneider E, Whitmore S, Glynn MK, et al. Revised surveillance case definitions for HIV infection among adults, adolescents, and children aged <18 months and for HIV infection and AIDS among children aged 18 months to <13 years—United States, 2008. MMWR 2008;57(RR10);1–8. Available at: www.cdc.gov/mmwr/preview/mmwrhtml/rr5710a1.htm. Accessed September 2, 2016.

acute HIV infection. Unfortunately, average time to receive these results in many centers is 7 to 14 days and may delay diagnosis. Patients with ARS may present with an OI in 20% to 25% of cases.

Respiratory disease

- *Pneumocystis jiroveci* pneumonia (PJP)
- Mycobacterial or fungal infections
- Sinusitis, bronchitis, or community-acquired pneumonia

Many common respiratory diseases in the general population are more common and sometimes more severe in HIV-positive patients, regardless of CD4 count. Infections include *Streptococcus pneumoniae* and *Haemophilus influenzae*, which commonly cause sinusitis, bronchitis, and pneumonia. For this reason, it is a general

Box 1
Acquired immunodeficiency syndrome–defining conditions

- Bacterial infections, multiple or recurrent[a]
- Candidiasis of bronchi, trachea, or lungs
- Candidiasis of esophagus[b]
- Cervical cancer, invasive[c]
- Coccidioidomycosis, disseminated or extrapulmonary
- Cryptococcosis, extrapulmonary
- Cryptosporidiosis, chronic intestinal (>1 month's duration)
- Cytomegalovirus disease (other than liver, spleen, or nodes), onset at age greater than 1 month
- Cytomegalovirus retinitis (with loss of vision)[b]
- Encephalopathy, HIV related
- Herpes simplex: chronic ulcers (>1 month's duration) or bronchitis, pneumonitis, or esophagitis (onset at age >1 month)
- Histoplasmosis, disseminated or extrapulmonary
- Isosporiasis, chronic intestinal (>1 month's duration)
- Kaposi sarcoma[b]
- Lymphoid interstitial pneumonia or pulmonary lymphoid hyperplasia complex[a,b]
- Lymphoma, Burkitt (or equivalent term)
- Lymphoma, immunoblastic (or equivalent term)
- Lymphoma, primary, of brain
- *Mycobacterium avium* complex or *Mycobacterium kansasii*, disseminated or extrapulmonary[b]
- *Mycobacterium tuberculosis* of any site, pulmonary[b,c], disseminated[b], or extrapulmonary[b]
- *Mycobacterium*, other species or unidentified species, disseminated[b] or extrapulmonary[b]
- *Pneumocystis jirovecii* pneumonia[b]
- Pneumonia, recurrent[b,c]
- Progressive multifocal leukoencephalopathy
- Salmonella septicemia, recurrent
- Toxoplasmosis of brain, onset at age greater than 1 month[b]
- Wasting syndrome attributed to HIV

[a] Only among children aged less than 13 years.
[b] Condition that might be diagnosed presumptively.
[c] Only among adults and adolescents aged greater than 13 years.
Adapted from CDC AIDS Defining Conditions 2008; *From* CDC. 1994 Revised classification system for human immunodeficiency virus infection in children less than 13 years of age. MMWR 1994;43;RR-12; CDC. 1993 Revised classification system for HIV infection and expanded surveillance case definition for AIDS among adolescents and adults. MMWR 1992;41:RR-17; and AIDS-Defining Conditions. MMWR Appendix A 2008;57(RR10):9. Available at: http://www.cdc.gov/mmwr/preview/mmwrhtml/rr5710a2.htm. Accessed September 2, 2016.

recommendation that all HIV-positive individuals receive both Pneumovax (PPV-23) and Prevnar (PCV13) pneumonia vaccines.[5,18]

PJP (formerly PCP) most often occurs when the CD4 count is less than 200 and in patients who have a previous diagnosis of PJP. Although cases of PJP have decreased dramatically due to ART and PJP prophylaxis, it is still the most common opportunistic cause of pneumonia in HIV-positive patients. Approximately half of the annual cases of PJP are made in patients who were not aware of their HIV status wherein PJP is the presenting illness.[19]

The clinical presentation of PJP includes fever, nonproductive cough, shortness of breath, retrosternal chest pain, low O_2 saturation, and unexplained weight loss. The onset of symptoms can be acute or indolent and worsen gradually over a period of weeks. Chest radiograph may appear normal (common in early disease), with faint bilateral interstitial infiltrates or ground-glass appearance on chest computed tomography. Laboratory data may show mild leukocytosis and LDH elevation.[5]

The preferred therapy for PJP infection is high-dose trimethoprim-sulfamethoxazole (TMP-SMX) double strength for 21 days with corticosteroids if Pao_2 is less than 70 mm Hg.[19,20] Alternate therapies include dapsone/trimethoprim or clindamycin/primaquine for patients with allergy or adverse events. The initial treatment phase should always be followed by secondary prophylaxis, preferably with TMP-SMX 1 tablet daily or dapsone 100 mg daily or atovoquone 1500 mg daily. Patients should be tested for G6PD deficiency before taking dapsone because hemolytic anemia is a potential side effect.[20] All patients with a CD4 count less than 200 or history of PJP should remain on PJP prophylaxis until the VL remains fully suppressed and CD4 count is greater than 200 for 3 to 6 months.[19]

Mycobacterium avium-intracellulare and Mycobacterium avium complex (MAC) are organisms that are ubiquitous in the environment and cause pulmonary and disseminated infections in severely immunocompromised patients. Exposure is thought to occur via inhalation or ingestion. Occurrence in AIDS patients with CD4 less than 50 is 20% to 40%, and these patients should be given chemoprophylaxis with azithromycin 1200 mg weekly.[19]

Other respiratory infections associated with HIV disease are Mycobacterium tuberculosis, and less commonly, fungal infections such as Aspergillus and Histoplasmosis.

Oropharyngeal and gastrointestinal disease

- Oral thrush (candidiasis)
- Hairy leukoplakia
- Apthous ulcers

Oral candidal infections may be minimally symptomatic, but can progress to esophageal candidiasis, which typically presents with retrosternal pain, odynophagia, weight loss, and medication intolerance. Treatment with fluconazole 100 to 200 mg daily for 7 to 14 days is suggested, depending on the severity and the level of immune suppression.

Herpes simplex virus (HSV) can cause oral or esophageal lesions, which can be painful and interfere with eating and swallowing medication. Valacyclovir 1000 to 2000 mg orally twice a day, acyclovir 400 mg upto 5 times a day[20] or famciclovir 500 mg orally twice a day may be used for treatment.[20] Duration of therapy may depend on severity and CD4 count.

Cytomegalovirus and MAC can cause gastritis, colitis, and diarrhea as well as cholecystitis.

Diarrhea is common in HIV and can be caused by opportunistic pathogens or direct effects of the virus. The clinical presentation is often with abdominal pain, diarrhea, fever, and weight loss. Bacterial pathogens such as *Salmonella, Shigella*, and *Campylobacter* can cause moderate to severe illness in HIV, and patients have higher risk of bacterial translocation from the gut in untreated HIV. *Salmonella typhi* infections can be up to 20 times more common in untreated HIV, and illness may be more severe.[5] The most common protozoal infections in HIV/AIDS are *Cryptosporidia, Microsporidia*, and *Isospora*. Although incidence of protozoal infections is low in the United States, workup for diarrhea in an immunocompromised patient should always include evaluation for ova and parasites. In patients who have recently received antibiotics, screening for *Clostridium difficile* should also be done.[5]

Liver disease

All HIV patients should be screened for hepatitis B virus (HBV) and hepatitis C virus (HCV) because these viruses are often acquired in the same way as HIV. Although infectious hepatitis is not considered an OI, HIV can be accelerated by and cause exacerbation of both hepatitis B and C. Because HBV is effectively treated by some HIV drugs, it is important to include 2 active HBV drugs in the HIV regimen.[17] Patients with chronic HBV infection should be reminded to continue safe sex in order to prevent transmission of both HIV and HBV because HBV is highly infectious.

Evidence of resolution of active HBV infection is demonstrated by loss of hepatitis B surface antigen and development of hepatitis B surface AB. The presence of hepatitis B surface AB confers immunity to the virus and will prevent reinfection. All HIV-positive patients who are not immune to HBV should be offered vaccination.[5,18]

Hepatitis C coinfection is 5% to 50% depending on risk factors and geographic location. The incidence is highest in injection drug users, and outbreaks of both infections have been increasing since 2014 with the resurgence of injection drug use and opioid addiction.

The development of direct-acting antivirals (DAAs) has increased the cure rates for HCV to close to 100% for all genotype 1 patients, with comparable cure rates in HIV patients. In HIV patients on ARV therapy, it is important to evaluate for possible drug-drug interactions with the HCV DAAs, and patients may require a change in their HIV medications in order to proceed with treatment.[17] Although an HCV-infected patient will develop AB to HCV, this does not confer immunity, and a patient who has either cleared HCV spontaneously or has posttreatment with DAAs may be reinfected with HCV.

Hepatitis A is less commonly encountered in the United States; however, there is an increased risk in MSM, and it is recommended that HIV-positive MSM receive the hepatitis A vaccine[18] (see Recommended Adult Immunization Schedule—United States—2016. Available at: http://www.cdc.gov/vaccines/schedules/downloads/adult/adult-schedule.pdf).

Genitourinary disease

Renal disease is common in HIV patients due to either opportunistic, comorbid infections or iatrogenic effect of medications used to treat HIV and OIs. HIV virus itself can have deleterious effects on the kidney and result in HIV-associated nephropathy (HIVAN). HIVAN is associated with proteinuria, enlarged hyperechoic kidneys, hypertension, and edema in severe disease. Diagnosis is confirmed with a biopsy specimen showing focal segmental glomerular sclerosis or mesangial proliferation. Almost 90% of cases of HIVAN are reported in African Americans, and clinical manifestations in this population are more severe and more often lead to renal failure.[5] All patients with signs of HIVAN should be initiated on ARV therapy with attention to choosing a renal friendly regimen of both ARVs and OI medications.[17]

All HIV patients should be screened for urethritis and urinary tract infections. Most often infections are related to comorbid STI, such as chlamydia, gonorrhea, syphilis, and HSV. It is important to identify and treat any STI promptly in order to reduce the risk of both STI and HIV transmission.[17]

Women with AIDS may develop severe vulvovaginal candidiasis if they have immune suppression and may require systemic treatment with fluconazole for resolution of symptoms.

Endocrine disease
Dyslipidemia is common in HIV patients treated with ART, and it is important to monitor lipid levels in all patients. Patients should be counseled on diet and exercise and evaluated for coronary artery disease risk to determine if lipid-lowering therapy is indicated. Drug interactions between ART therapy and many statins are common; however, rosuvastatin and atorvastatin can be used safely at lower doses.[21]

Neurologic disease
Neurologic OIs are much less common in the post-ART era but are still seen as presenting illness in AIDS diagnoses.

Toxoplasmosis is an OI caused by a parasite commonly found in undercooked meat. About 15% of Americans have antibodies to Toxoplasma, and infection in AIDS is most commonly related to reactivation of latent tissue cysts. It is the most common central nervous system (CNS) -related OI and clinical presentation includes fever, headache, and focal neurologic deficits. All AIDS patients should be screened for IgG AB to toxoplasmosis because infection is 10% more likely in AB-positive patients.[5]

Cryptococcal meningitis is another important CNS-related OI that presents with fever, headache, nausea/vomiting, altered mental status, neck rigidity, and visual changes. Opening pressure is often elevated on lumbar puncture (LP) and at times serial LP may be necessary to lower pressures. Diagnosis is made by identification of cryptococcal antigen in the cerebrospinal fluid (CSF). Therapy for cryptococcus should initially be with intravenous amphotericin B and flucytosine until CSF studies are negative. Then the patient may be transitioned to fluconazole to complete 8 weeks of treatment dosing at 400 mg per day. Secondary prophylaxis for Cryptococcus should continue at 200 mg daily until the CD4 count is safely greater than 200 for 6 months.[19,20] Although in general it is recommended to start ART quickly after diagnosis of HIV disease, in patients with Cryptococcal meningitis it is recommended that ART be delayed until approximately 2 to 4 weeks after clearance of Cryptococcus from the CSF in order to avoid recurrent cryptococcal disease if there is a rapid increase in CD4 count and immune reconstitution inflammatory syndrome.[5,19]

ANTIRETROVIRAL THERAPY—WHEN TO START

Patients with recent OI or CD4 count less than 200 should be started on ART urgently with the exception of Cryptococcal meningitis, where therapy should be delayed 2 to 4 weeks or until there is confirmation of clearance of Cryptococcus from the CSF.[5,19] Since 2012, it has been recommended that ART be started on all HIV-positive individuals, regardless of CD4 count or time since infection. Studies including the SMART trial showed significant benefit in morbidity and mortality in patients continuously on ART compared with those with similar CD4 counts that were randomized to discontinue ART with close monitoring of CD4 level.[15] Treating all infected patients also aims to decrease rates of transmission especially in recently infected patients. Decreasing the number of patients in a community with uncontrolled viremia decreases the "community viral load," which is part of the strategy of TasP.[2]

Newer ART options have much less toxicity and lower pill burden, including many STR, which are dosed once daily. Patient education regarding the importance of adherence to avoid drug resistance and complications, discussion of lifestyle, dietary habits, and use of other medications is essential for successful therapy. Many combinations of ART could potentially cause drug-drug interactions, which may inhibit absorption of medications or cause toxicity for the patient. In cases where there is concern for clinical complication or psychosocial issues that may limit the ability to achieve effective viral control, ART may be delayed until concerns can be addressed. Ultimately, all patients engaged in care should be on ART.[17]

ANTIRETROVIRAL THERAPY—WHAT TO START

Traditionally, ART has consisted of at least 3 active drugs against HIV, determined by genotype testing, which may identify any naive drug resistance mutations. It is recommended that all patients have genotype testing at entry to care and again if sufficient time has passed between initial genotype and initiation of ART. Most regimens consist of at least 2 nucleoside reverse transcriptase inhibitors (NRTI) and one drug from another class, such as nonnucleoside reverse transcriptase inhibitor (NNRTI), protease inhibitor (PI), or integrase strand transfer inhibitor (INSTI) (Table 4). When possible,

---

Table 4
Recommended, Alternative, and Other Antiretroviral Regimen Options for Treatment-Naive Patients

Recommended Regimen Options

Recommended regimens are those with demonstrated durable virologic efficacy, favorable tolerability and toxicity profiles, and ease of use.

INSTI plus 2-NRTI Regimen:
- DTG/ABC/3TC[a] (AI)—if HLA-B*5701 negative
- DTG plus either TDF/FTC[a] (AI) or TAF/FTC[b] (AII)
- EVG/c/TAF/FTC (AI) or EVG/c/TDF/FTC (AI)
- RAL plus either TDF/FTC[a] (AI) or TAF/FTC[b] (AII)

Boosted PI plus 2 NRTIs:
- DRV/r plus either TDF/FTC[a] (AI) or TAF/FTC[b] (AII)

Alternative Regimen Options

Alternative regimens are effective and tolerable, but have potential disadvantages when compared with the Recommended regimens, have limitations for use in certain patient populations, or have less supporting data from randomized clinical trials. **However, an Alternative regimen may be the preferred regimen for some patients.**

NNRTI plus 2 NRTIs:
- EFV/TDF/FTC[a] (BI)
- EFV plus TAF/FTC[b] (BII)
- RPV/TDF/FTC[a] (BI) or RPV/TAF/FTC[b] (BII)—if HIV RNA <100,000 copies/mL and CD4 >200 cells/mm³

Boosted PI plus 2 NRTIs:
- (ATV/c or ATV/r) plus either TDF/FTC[a] (BI) or TAF/FTC[b] (BII)
- DRV/c (BIII) or DRV/r (BII) plus ABC/3TC[a]—if HLA-B*5701 negative
- DRV/c plus either TDF/FTC[a] (BII) or TAF/FTC[b] (BII)

[a] 3TC may be substituted for FTC, or vice versa, if a non-fixed dose NRTI combination is desired.
[b] The evidence supporting this regimen is based on relative bioavailability data coupled with data from randomized, controlled switch trials demonstrating the safety and efficacy of TAF-containing regimens.

Adapted from Guidelines for the use of antiretroviral agents in HIV-1-infected adults and adolescents. Available at: https://aidsinfo.nih.gov/contentfiles/lvguidelines/AA_Tables.pdf; with permission. Accessed September 2, 2016.

it is recommended to use an STR, which is a complete 3- to 4-drug regimen in one pill dosed once daily. In the spring of 2015, significant changes were made to the Department of Health and Human Services (DHHS) guidelines[17] in regards to preferred ART regimens. The first STR and commonly used medication (FTC/tenofovir/efavirenz [EFV] combination) was removed from the recommended therapy list due to high occurrence of CNS side effects.

ANTIRETROVIRAL DRUG CLASSES/SPECIFIC DRUGS
Nucleoside/Nucleotide Reverse Transcriptase Inhibitors

These drugs block the replication of the viral particle at the point of the RNA-dependent DNA synthesis (see "The HIV Life Cycle" infographic at: https://aidsinfo.nih.gov/education-materials/fact-sheets/19/73/the-hivlife-cycle), and typically, 2 drugs from this class are used as a basis of an ART regimen.

Today the drugs lamivudine (3TC) or FTC are included in nearly all HIV regimens due to their low toxicity and general effectiveness as well as being effective against HBV. Note these drugs are similar in chemical structure and should not be used together.

Tenofovir disoproxil fumarate (TDF) has been used as a second NRTI in most ART regimens and is available in multiple STRs. TDF is also effective against hepatitis B and should be used along with either FTC or 3TC as combination therapy for patients coinfected with hepatitis B. TDF may cause renal side effects, decreased bone mineral density, and increased incidence of avascular necrosis of the joints. A newer version of tenofovir, now tenofovir alafenamide fumarate (TAF), has recently been approved, and studies show this drug has higher intracellular levels and much less renal toxicity and deleterious effect on bone mineral density.[17]

Abacavir (ABC) is another commonly used NRTI and is also dosed in combination with FTC or 3TC and an agent from another class as part of a once-daily ART regimen. ABC may cause a severe hypersensitivity reaction, which can be fatal if the drug is continued. All patients who may be started on ABC should be screened for HLA B-5701, which, if positive, predicts hypersensitivity, and patients who are positive should not receive ABC. Signs of ABC-related hypersensitivity include fever, rash, nausea, and vomiting. Patients who have negative HLA testing can take ABC without concern, although they should continue to be monitored closely.

The first HIV drug zidovudine (AZT) is still included in drug regimens in specific instances, especially in prevention of perinatal HIV infection. Other older drugs in this class, including stavudine and didanosine, have been implicated in lipodystrophy/lipoatrophy syndrome as well as peripheral neuropathy and are not generally recommended.[17]

Nonnucleoside Reverse Transcriptase Inhibitors

These drugs block the virus at a slightly different location than NRTIs and specifically inhibit DNA polymerization (see "The HIV Life Cycle" infographic at: https://aidsinfo.nih.gov/education-materials/fact-sheets/19/73/the-hivlife-cycle), which is essential for viral replication. EFV was widely used as part of the first STR regimen along with TDF and FTC for many years. This drug is generally well tolerated but commonly causes abnormal dreams and CNS side effects. With wider use, it was found to be associated with higher incidence of depression and suicide.

First-generation NNRTIs have a lower barrier to resistance, where one mutation may render the drugs ineffective and breakthrough viremia will result, placing the patient at risk for additional mutations to the other drugs in the regimen as well as increased risk for HIV transmission. NNRTI resistance mutations tend to persist for longer than mutations to other antiretroviral classes and have been identified in patients who are naive to ART.

Second-generation NNRTIs etravirine (ETR) and rilpivirine (RPV) are often still effective in the setting of the common mutations and in general are well tolerated.

RPV is available in an STR with TDF or TAF and FTC and is commonly used; however, there is a warning to avoid use of RPV in patients with HIV VL >100,000 due to decreased effectiveness in this group. ETR is most commonly used in patients with a history of more extensive drug resistance or other tolerability issues because this drug must be dosed twice a day. Common side effects across this class include rash, nausea, and hepatotoxicity.[17]

Nevaripine is still widely used in Africa. Recent warnings about increased incidence of hepatotoxicity in women over age 35 have also made providers cautious about choosing this drug in a regimen.

Protease Inhibitors

These drugs work by blocking the formation of proteins used in the maturation of the virus just before the viral particles bud off and are released from the cell (see "The HIV Life Cycle" infographic at: https://aidsinfo.nih.gov/education-materials/fact-sheets/19/73/the-hivlife-cycle). The introduction of PIs in the 1990s changed the tide of the AIDS epidemic because these agents used in combination with NRTIs could fully suppress viral replication to less than 500 copies of virus per microliter, and there was a rapid decline in AIDS-related deaths. Early PIs caused frequent side effects, including dyslipidemia, gastrointestinal upset, and nephrolithiasis. Ritonavir, one of the earliest PIs to be developed, is not well tolerated at treatment doses but is still used widely as a booster of other PIs in order to decrease pill burden and dosing frequency. Drug interactions are very common with ritonavir as it is a strong CYP3A4 inhibitor and providers should use care in prescribing other drugs to patients on any PI.

The recommended first-line PI in a treatment-naive patient is darunavir (DRV) boosted with ritonavir, and as an alternative, atazanavir (ATV) boosted with ritonavir. DRV is generally well tolerated, although skin rash may occur and at times may be severe and related to the sulfonamide moiety of the compound; however, many sulfonamide allergic patients will tolerate DRV without rash. ATV may cause hyperbilirubinemia without elevation of liver function tests. ATV may cause icterus and jaundice in some patients, which is a common reason for discontinuation.

Older PIs, such as lopinavir/ritonavir, and fosamprenavir are still commonly used but no longer recommended as first line.[17]

Fusion and Entry Inhibitors

These drugs block the binding/fusion of HIV to the CD4 cell, preventing the virus from entering the cell (see "The HIV Life Cycle" infographic at: https://aidsinfo.nih.gov/education-materials/fact-sheets/19/73/the-hivlife-cycle).

Enfuvirtide blocks virus entry by preventing fusion of the virus to the cell by binding the gp41 region of the HIV envelope. This drug is only available in injection form, is dosed twice daily, and commonly causes injection site reactions, and therefore, it is not commonly used.

Miraviroc (MVC) is a CCR5 receptor antagonist that blocks the binding of the virus to the CD4 cell. MVC is indicated only for patients that are CCR5 receptor positive, and a trophile assay to determine the tropism of the CD4 cell should be completed before initiating treatment. Patients whose trophile assay shows X4 receptors or dual/mixed tropism (CCR5/X4) should not use this medication.

Integrase Strand Transfer Inhibitors

Integrase inhibitors are the newest class of HIV drugs and work by inhibition of the enzyme that is used to insert the proviral DNA particle into the host cell genome (see "The HIV Life Cycle" infographic at: https://aidsinfo.nih.gov/education-materials/fact-sheets/19/73/the-hivlife-cycle). Raltegravir (RAL) is generally very well tolerated with minimal adverse effects and drug interactions. Elvitegravir (EVG) is available as an STR (EVG/cobisistat [COBI]/TDF/FTC or EVG/COBI/TAF/FTC) and is boosted with a novel boosting agent COBI. COBI is also a strong CYP3A4 inhibitor and may cause similar drug interactions to ritonavir. Dolutegravir (DTG) is the newest INSTI and is very potent with small pill size, once-daily dosing, low incidence of side effects, and minimal drug interactions. Studies have shown very rapid time to full viral suppression in patients with DTG-containing regimens and overall low incidence of drug-resistance mutations with this drug.[17] DTG is available in a STR (DTG/3TC/ABC) and is recommended as first-line therapy for ART-naive patients.

HUMAN IMMUNODEFICIENCY VIRUS AND PREGNANCY

Discussion regarding childbearing intentions and pregnancy planning, including healthy lifestyle, safer sex, and contraception options, should be discussed throughout the care of the woman with HIV. Patients interested in hormonal contraception should initiate these therapies; however, drug-drug interactions should be taken into account. Patients contemplating pregnancy should have medications adjusted to achieve full viral suppression and discontinuation of any potentially teratogenic agents. HIV-positive women who become pregnant should be initiated on ART as soon as possible, even before results of genotype testing because studies have shown that earlier time to viral suppression decreases rate of perinatal HIV transmission. Combined intrapartum, antepartum, and infant antiretroviral prophylaxis is recommended because antiretroviral drugs reduce perinatal transmission by several mechanisms, including lowering maternal VL and providing infant PrEP and PEP. VL monitoring should be performed at baseline, 1 month after initiation, and every 3 months once the she becomes undetectable, and at approximately 34 to 36 weeks' gestation to guide planning for method of delivery. Women should be counseled about the risks and benefits of medications, including ART and other OI prophylaxis medications if necessary. Intrapartum use of intravenous AZT and cesarean delivery may be recommended if there is concern for VL >1000/mL. Most infants will receive postnatal AZT prophylaxis for 4 to 6 weeks depending on the exposure history.[12]

SUMMARY

HIV continues to spread worldwide, and in the United States, HIV disproportionately affects African Americans and MSM. At-risk individuals should be identified, and those who test positive should be linked to care and initiated on ART as soon as possible. Early diagnosis and treatment significantly reduce the incidence of OIs and are key to the public health efforts to implement treatment as prevention to help reduce new infection rates in high-risk populations. Advances in ART have made medications more tolerable and resulted in improved survival rates and less drug toxicity. PrEP is an effective therapy that may reduce the risk of HIV infection and should be offered to individuals at high risk for HIV exposure. Universal HIV screening in pregnancy and rapid initiation of ART for pregnant women, as well as intrapartum ART, has reduced the perinatal infection rate in the United States dramatically.

REFERENCES

1. HIV in the United States: at a glance. Centers for Disease Control and Prevention Web site. Available at: www.cdc.gov/hiv/statistics/overview/ataglance.html. Accessed June 26, 2016.
2. HIV Care Continuum. AIDS.gov Web site. 2015. Available at: https://www.aids.gov/federal-resources/policies/care-continuum/. Accessed June 26, 2016.
3. Centers for Disease Control and Prevention. Revised recommendations for HIV testing of adults, adolescents, and pregnant women in health-care settings. MMWR Recomm Rep 2006;55:1–17.
4. Global AIDS Update 2016. UNAIDS Web site. 2016. Available at: http://www.unaids.org/en/resources/documents/2016/Global-AIDS-update-2016. Accessed June 26, 2016.
5. Fauci AS, Lane HC. Human immunodeficiency virus disease: AIDS and related disorders. In: Kasper DL, Fauci AS, editors. Harrison's infectious diseases. 2nd edition. New York: McGraw-Hill Education; 2013. p. 842–942.
6. 10 million men stepped up for HIV prevention. World Health Organization Web site. 2015. Available at: http://apps.who.int/iris/bitstream/10665/202249/1/WHO_HIV_2015.50_eng.pdf?ua=1. Accessed June 26, 2016.
7. Hormonal contraception and the risk of HIV acquisition in women. World Health Organization Web site. 2016. Available at: http://www.who.int/reproductivehealth/topics/family_planning/statement/en/. Accessed June 26, 2016.
8. Heffron R, Donnell D, Rees H, et al. Use of hormonal contraceptives and risk of HIV-1 transmission: a prospective cohort study. Lancet Infect Dis 2012;12(1):19–26.
9. Centers for Disease Control and Prevention and Association of Public Health Laboratories. Laboratory testing for the diagnosis of HIV infection: updated recommendations. 2014. Available at: http://dx.doi.org/10.15620/cdc.23447. Accessed June 26, 2016.
10. US Public Health Service. Preexposure prophylaxis for the prevention of HIV infection in the United States—2014: A clinical practice guideline. Available at: http://www.cdc.gov/hiv/pdf/guidelines/PrEPguidelines2014.pdf. Accessed June 28, 2016.
11. Molina JM, Capitant C, Spire B, et al. On-demand preexposure prophylaxis in men at high risk for HIV-1 infection. N Engl J Med 2015;373:2237–46.
12. Panel on treatment of HIV-infected pregnant women and prevention of perinatal transmission. Recommendations for use of antiretroviral drugs in pregnant HIV-1-infected women for maternal health and interventions to reduce perinatal HIV transmission in the United States. Available at: http://aidsinfo.nih.gov/contentfiles/lvguidelines/PerinatalGL.pdf. Accessed June 28, 2016.
13. Centers for Disease Control and Prevention and U.S. Department of Health and Human Services. Updated guidelines for antiretroviral postexposure prophylaxis after sexual, injection drug use, or other nonoccupational exposure to HIV—United States, 2016. Available at: https://stacks.cdc.gov/view/cdc/38856. Accessed June 28, 2016.
14. AIDS defining conditions. Centers for Disease Control and Prevention. 2008. Available at: http://www.cdc.gov/mmwr/preview/mmwrhtml/rr5710a2.htm. Accessed June 26, 2016.

15. The Strategies for Management of Antiretroviral Therapy (SMART) Study Group. CD4+ count-guided interruption of antiretroviral treatment. N Engl J Med 2006; 355(22):2283–96.
16. May MT, Vehreschild JJ, Trickey A, et al. Mortality according to CD4 count at start of combination antiretroviral therapy among HIV-infected patients followed for up to 15 years after start of treatment: collaborative cohort study. Clin Infect Dis 2016;62(12):1571–7.
17. Panel on Antiretroviral Guidelines for Adults and Adolescents. Guidelines for the use of antiretroviral agents in HIV-1-infected adults and adolescents. Bethesda (MD): NIH, Department of Health and Human Services. Available at: http://www.aidsinfo.nih.gov/ContentFiles/AdultandAdolescentGL.pdf. Accessed April 1, 2016.
18. Recommended adult immunization schedule—United States—2016. Centers for Disease Control and Prevention Web site. 2016. Available at: http://www.cdc.gov/vaccines/schedules/downloads/adult/adult-schedule.pdf. Accessed June 28, 2016.
19. Panel on Opportunistic Infections in HIV-Infected Adults and Adolescents. Guidelines for the prevention and treatment of opportunistic infections in HIV-infected adults and adolescents: recommendations from the Centers for Disease Control and Prevention, the National Institutes of Health, and the HIV Medicine Association of the Infectious Diseases Society of America. Available at: http://aidsinfo.nih.gov/contentfiles/lvguidelines/adult_oi.pdf. Accessed August 31, 2016.
20. Glibert DM, Chambers HF, Eliopoulos GM, et al. The Sanford guide to antimicrobial therapy. 46th edition. 2016.
21. Feinstein MJ, Axhenbach CJ, Stone NJ, et al. A systemic review of the usefulness of statin therapy in HIV-infected patients. Am J Cardiol 2015;115(12):1760–6.

Printed and bound by CPI Group (UK) Ltd, Croydon, CR0 4YY

07/10/2024

01040504-0020